D0729188

THE GARAGE GYM

ATHLETE

THE PRACTICAL GUIDE TO TRAINING LIKE A PRO, UNLEASHING FITNESS FREEDOM, AND LIVING THE SIMPLE LIFE

By Jerred Moon

Copyright © 2016 Jerred Moon

Publishing by:

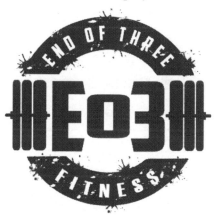

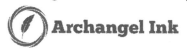

www.EndofThreeFitness.com

Publishing Services Provided by

Archangel Ink

ISBN: 10:1530178452

ISBN-13: 978-1530178452

Dedication:

Nothing I do would be possible without my wife, Emily. I love you more and more each day. *Sic Parvis Magna.*

To my sons, you are two incredible human beings. Pursue your passion with an unrelenting work ethic and you will find happiness. Don't chase shiny objects; your happiness will come from the pursuit itself.

Disclaimer:

This book provides multiple do-it-yourself (DIY) projects. As with any do-it-yourself project, unfamiliarity with the tools and process can be dangerous. Projects in this book should be viewed as entertainment only. End of Three Fitness and the creators, will not be held responsible for any injury due to the misuse or misunderstanding of any DIY project. All DIY projects are purely "at your own risk." If you are at all uncomfortable or inexperienced working on projects yourself (especially projects involving dangerous tools), please reconsider doing the job yourself. It is very possible on any DIY to damage your property, create a hazardous condition, harm, or even kill yourself or others.

All information in this book is for education and entertainment purposes only. End of Three Fitness and its employees (End of Three Fitness Enterprises, LLC.), as well as any partnering websites, are not liable for any damages that arise out of your access to our books or websites, whether they be direct, indirect, special, incidental, consequential, or punitive.

Information and recommendations given by End of Three Fitness, and the creator, (End of Three Fitness Enterprises, LLC.) are not intended as a substitute for the medical advice and treatment of a doctor. The content of this book is intended for general use and is not designed to diagnose or treat medical conditions or to replace medical advice.

Note from the Author

Hey there, Garage Gym Athlete! Jerred Moon here, founder of End of Three Fitness, a website designed to make you a better human. End of Three Fitness has been awarded multiple "Top Fitness Blog" titles, has been featured in magazines, and has amassed millions of visitors from all around the world since its launch at the end of 2011.

Since its inception, the backbone to End of Three Fitness has truly been all the information and articles about garage gyms, and helping people succeed in this arena has been an amazing journey. I am excited you are considering joining this revolution.

Garage Gym Athlete will provide you with a complete guide to creating your own garage gym. But I want it to do way more than that. I want this book to fire you up, to show you some tips and tricks I've gathered from coaching over the years, and to give you more autonomy in your health and fitness.

If this book does its job, then I will be looking forward to meeting you at Garage Gym Athlete, the #1 Garage Gym community in the world.

We have workouts, programs, courses, and more to help you crush this whole garage gym thing. Sign up to be a part of our community at:

- GarageGymAthlete.com

For more details about Garage Gym Athlete and your special gift for purchasing the Garage Gym Athlete book...read below:

Garage Gym Athlete is made up of three components:

1. Daily Workouts

2. A Thriving Community

3. Training Programs

Garage Gym Athlete provides the highest quality programming at the best price you will find, and it is 100 percent catered to the minimalist garage gym exerciser. Join our community and get stronger, faster and harder to kill!

Garage Gym Athlete SPECIAL for *Garage Gym Athlete* readers ONLY:

For a limited time, we are offering a HUGE discount to *you* on a Garage Gym Athlete Membership. To join now, go here: GarageGymAthlete.com and enter promo code: **'REVOLUTION'**: and let's start this revolution! Are you ready!?

Well, are you ready to get extremely fit, at home? Are you ready for a garage gym? It is time to take a stand. It is time get rid of all the supplements that don't work and that you don't need, time to trade in the crazy-expensive gym memberships, and throw away the fitness magazines that push useless products and programs designed for people who aren't you.

It is time to start making some decisions for yourself, and decisions affecting your health should not be taken lightly. Thomas Jefferson put it this way: "Leave all the afternoon for exercise and recreation, which are as necessary as reading. I will rather say more necessary because health is worth more than learning."

Good luck on your garage gym journey!

Table of Contents

Section One

Fitness Freedom

Chapter 1

What is a Garage Gym Athlete?

If you have a body, you are an athlete.

—Bill Bowerman, Nike co-founder

So, you're thinking about starting a garage gym? Good idea!

Seriously, the grassroots movement that is garage gyms is exploding for a number of reasons, and I am truly excited for you to begin your journey, so let's dive right in.

Are you sick of all that is involved with getting in shape—with becoming stronger and fitter?

Training and getting in shape can be a chore at times, but is it really the training you don't enjoy? With a little observation, or self-analysis, you may find the chore is often not the training itself. Of course, you may not love to exercise, but is it really that bad?

The worst part about fitness is all that comes with it: a long commute to the gym, crowds of people, occupied equipment, hygiene concerns, monthly fees, and much more. You have a job, family, and all of life's chores and tasks to worry about. Who wants to start or end their day with what feels like another chore? A trip to the gym involves changing into appropriate clothes, driving, waiting, more driving . . . and the routine simply takes you from one climate-controlled box (work) to another (the gym) with your only chance for fresh air coming from walking across the parking lot. Not to mention that every day you "just don't feel like it" and decide to skip the gym, it costs you money!

Commercial gyms are designed for the masses—TVs, isolation machines, and a bunch of stuff you don't really need. It may make you feel better to have "gone to the gym today" but wouldn't you rather train effectively and efficiently? Your head should be nodding at this point.

Perhaps when you think of a garage gym, you think of Rocky Balboa chasing chickens and lifting logs. Or maybe you think of a version of your commercial gym stuffed in your garage.

The reality is somewhere in between. A garage gym can be an effective and efficient world-class training facility. It is built to suit your performance. Some of the fittest people in the world train in garage gyms regularly because they know the secret: less equipment, fewer isolation exercises, and less junk; but more efficient training.

The thought that will eventually cross your mind is, "I don't have the money or time to make my own garage my gym." While certainly not dirt cheap, you can do it for as little as $500, which is the equivalent of about a year and a half of the cheapest gym pass. If you use your garage gym for just two years, you will have made money on the investment. In addition, it only takes about two weeks to complete. And that's if you take your time. And now is the time to become a Garage Gym Athlete.

In the past, it was near impossible to have a garage gym. Not too long ago you wouldn't be able to find a store that sold a kettlebell, and to order one online would have cost you a fortune in shipping fees. Not to mention any larger and heavier equipment you may need.

Currently, it is very affordable. Luckily, the popularity of CrossFit® and the sport of weight lifting have exploded in recent years. This popularity has made getting high-quality barbells, plates, and other equipment much more economical. There are plenty of stores and websites that offer free shipping and easy availability.

In the future, it will become even more affordable. And just a prediction here; when the supply of CrossFit® gyms exceeds the demand in coming years, you'll potentially see CrossFit® gyms going out of business left and right. Now, while I wish nothing bad upon any gym owner, or their livelihood, it will make for an opportunity for you to snag great equipment at huge discounts.

In spite of affordability, you have to be a little crazy to want to pursue fitness outside of the conventional gym, right?

Well, I don't think the Garage Gym Athlete is crazy, I consider the Garage Gym Athlete "other." A term I like to use a lot is the "other guy (and gal)" to describe those who are interested in becoming a Garage Gym Athlete. Never be average, always be other.

The other guy is not average; he is a doer. If it can make him better, he'll try it. If it's too heavy, he'll learn how to lift it. If it's too far, he'll still run to it. He will take on many challenges, is comfortable with the fact that things will never be perfect, and will go out knowing he was never average.

Life Happens.

Maybe you got stuck in a desk. Maybe your schedule got filled to the brim. Maybe you feel like an average life, for you, is like fitting a square peg into a round hole.

Well, if you're reading this, there's a good chance you would like to make some changes. You'd like to see how strong you can actually become, how fast you can truly run, and how much better you can actually be.

That's why End of Three Fitness exists! And to embrace being "other" is to be a Garage Gym Athlete.

Chapter 2

Why Be a Garage Gym Athlete?

Now, perhaps I am starting this book off a little too philosophical for some of you, but I've seen a lot of people go through this process and fail.

I'm truly passionate about making this stick in your life! To make something stick, we have to start with why.

Why are you, or do you want to be, a Garage Gym Athlete? Why work out in the cold, in hot, or in confined spaces? Why do you want to achieve what you want to achieve?

That is a very important question.

And one you *have* to be crystal clear on! To be honest; to not answer that question will eventually make you the guy who is selling your garage gym equipment for pennies on the dollar to the rest of us who did answer that question.

Let me share my story and perhaps it will help you.

Years ago, I decided to break up with the globo gyms of the world and pass on CrossFit® boxes. If you are scratching your head on the term "globo gym," it's essentially a typical large-sized gym in today's world.

Right after I got married, my wife and I were running up hill financially. Let's put it this way: strapped for cash, no savings, and living with my wife's parents.

I was going to be an officer in the Air Force, but had to wait till my active duty orders started. To make things crazier, my wife and I started day one of our marriage $100,000 in debt! Long story short—I was stressed out.

I was working odd jobs, making things work, and trying to squeeze fitness into the mix. I couldn't afford a globo gym, and a CrossFit® gym was out of the question because in most cases a CrossFit® affiliate is more expensive than a globo gym. I convinced my wife (she's awesome) to let me use some of our wedding money to buy a barbell and rubberized bumper plates.

In using our wedding money for gym equipment, there were only two realistic potential outcomes.

Outcome #1: I spend the money, I use the equipment religiously, and everyone is happy, because in the long run I am saving us money.

Outcome #2: I buy the equipment, the excitement fades, I stop working out in the garage. My wife thinks I'm an idiot, and I would be an idiot to spend what little money we had and *waste* it.

Right from the start, my "why" was to show my wife that I am the type of man that sticks to his word, who spends our money wisely, and doesn't quit anything.

I did not have the forethought at that time to have a "big why," but I luckily stumbled into having a gigantic "why" when I started my garage gym.

Maybe that sounds crazy, but my why was to show my wife the type of man I am. The best part is that "why" turned into a habit.

- Extreme heat—I got a fan.
- Freezing cold—I put on sweats.
- No space—I went outside.
- Not enough equipment—I made it work.

The "why" to me was so big, there was no quitting. There was no, "I don't feel like it," and that has made this whole Garage Gym Athlete thing really stick.

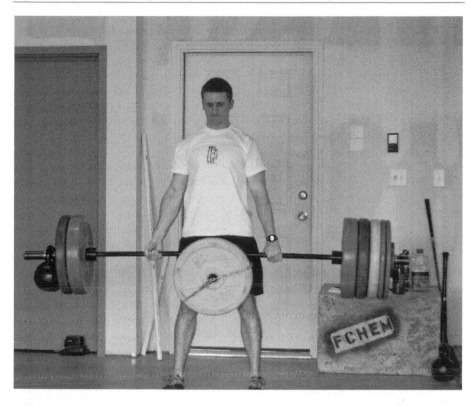

Believe me when I tell you it has not been easy. I am not writing this from the perspective of some guy who has all the time in the world.

When I really kicked things up in the garage gym, I was going through pilot training in the United States Air Force, which has one of the most demanding time tables in the U.S. military, and things never slowed down. Over the years, I worked *crazy* hours, my wife and I have added two children into the mix, and to be honest, at times, I don't know how I fit it all in.

I'll say it again, as a family man with real time constraints it has been challenging over the years. My motivation has gone on roller coaster rides, my programming has jumped all over the place, and I have seen my progress not only stall, but move backwards.

It will happen to you, and it's okay. Life will happen and you'll get sidetracked. Some event will come and knock you right off your feet.

But the only thing that is going to keep you coming back, embracing the elements, and working your butt off is to have a gigantic "why" that will see you through any struggle.

Now, it's your turn.

It's pretty simple. Just answer the following questions:

What is your goal?

-   Is it to lift 2½ times your body weight?

-   Is it to run a marathon?

-   Is it to compete in a CrossFit® competition?

-   Is it to lose weight?

-   Is it to gain muscle?

Why do you want that?

-   Why are you, or do you want to be, a Garage Gym Athlete?

-   Why work out in cold, hot, or confined spaces?

-   Why do you want to achieve what you want to achieve?

Remember, the *bigger* the better!

Once you've done this, you can move on to the next chapter and we will cover the greatest mistakes to avoid in being a Garage Gym Athlete.

Chapter 3

The Great Mistakes

My first garage gym was miserable!

We're talking dangerously hot.

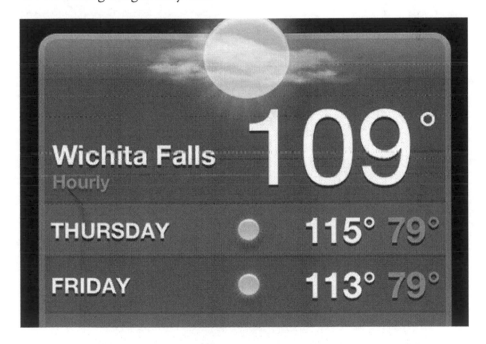

But it was incredibly fun!

Most of my garage gym was DIY, and so were my programs. I may have been honing in my skills as a carpenter, but the biggest skill I was refining each day was becoming a programmer. When you hear the term "programmer" in this book, it simply means structuring, writing, and planning workout programs and schedules.

Pre-garage gym, I was already writing programs and workouts. However, with a garage gym and minimal equipment I had to become even better at programming. I had to learn what was needed, what wasn't needed, and most importantly what actually worked!

But I'm getting ahead of myself here. In this chapter, I would like to lay out mistakes you can avoid, and the number one principle you can apply to see results.

If you did the exercise in the last chapter then you're super clear on what you want in being a Garage Gym Athlete, including your *big why*.

Now, the big question is *how can you get there*? How can you achieve the goal that you've set? Let me start by giving you a completely non-fitness related goal.

I'll tell you up front one of the best lessons I have ever learned is: Start and Stick. Meaning just freaking start and stick with it!

I mentioned previously that when my wife and I got married we collectively owed $100,000. Yes, $100K in debt right on the very first day of our marriage.

It wasn't stupid debt. We had two cars, thus we had car loans. We had just finished school and had student loans, and one little crazy incident with our dog and we now had medical debt—yes, from a dog.

And the grand total was $100,000.

My wife and I had decided that she would be a stay-at-home mom, but we had also decided we were going to commit, and do whatever we had to, to get out of debt. It was painful, stressful, and challenging. After we committed we slowly started to see our debt come down. Each month we were able to breathe just a little bit better. By breathe I mean our first budget gave us seventeen dollars of wiggle room each month. No mistakes allowed. But we made mistakes; we weren't perfect. We *did* start and we did stick to our goal.

Guess what? In just under three years after getting married, with a ton of discipline and with my salary as a military officer we paid off *all* of our debt! And we are now debt free!

Why do I share this? Because I've achieved fitness goals, business goals, and financial goals, and this simple principle applies to all of them.

Start and Stick!

Now, back to garage gyms. As long as you know starting and sticking will be the biggest things you can do in a garage gym then we can move to the smaller mistakes, which can still derail your progress.

Mistake #1: Too much emphasis on the "right" equipment.

If you think a lack of equipment is holding you back, you're wrong! I started with a barbell, some plates, and I built a set of DIY rings and a plyometric box. I *only* used those items for a long time and saw great results.

Thinking you need to start with a GHD (Glute Ham Developer) machine, Reverse Hyperextension machine, and Concept 2 rower is the wrong train of thought. If you've got the money, go for it! But I didn't so I built *everything*.

I would save up to do one DIY project at a time. I slowly built up an arsenal of DIY equipment, garage sale finds, and other goodies. This was my garage gym at the end of year one:

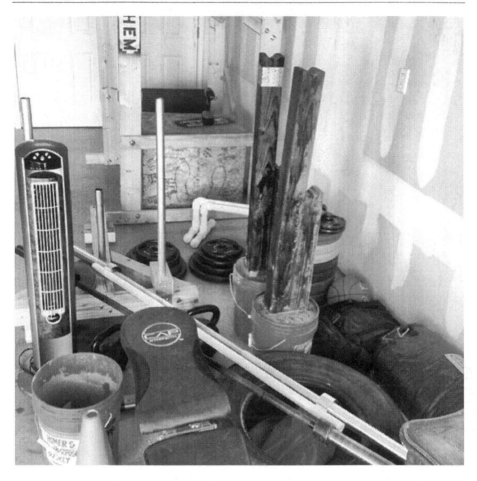

You can make it work with a lot less, and in a lot less space, which brings me to mistake number two.

Mistake #2: Getting discouraged about your space.

Being in the military gave me a unique opportunity to have around five different garage gym spaces:

- — Some were freezing cold.

- — Some were crazy hot.

- — Some were outside.

- — Some didn't give me enough space to press overhead.

   – Some were with the ground too slanted to lift with good form.

I've trained in all of them. Sometimes it sucked and I would get frustrated, but I would make it work.

I found ways to shove a barbell in a Honda Accord. I've traveled with kettlebells. I've done Olympic lifting in grass and dirt. I've hung rings on trees and under bridges. The takeaway: Make it work! If you can't change the space you have, find a way to make it work in your situation. Let me erase that excuse from your head right now. You *can* find the space.

Mistake #3: Trying to do everything by yourself.

Look, what I haven't told you is the whole time I was starting and using a garage gym, I was making a *huge* mistake. Sometimes I fall prey to superhero syndrome. Essentially that means I think I can do it all *alone* by

   – Building DIY projects

   – Doing my own programming

   – Trying to motivate myself

You'll only get so far that way. I've followed that path and things have probably been two times as hard and taken two times as long as they should have. You need accountability and direction from someone who has been where you are trying to go.

I know the garage gym can be a lonely place, but something as simple as sharing workouts with a friend (in a different part of the country) and comparing times at the end of the day can go a long way. I know because I've done it.

   – Who is helping you?

   – Who is holding you accountable?

If your answer is "no one," then stop and go get someone right now. It's *vital* to reaching your goal. We also have massive community at End of Three Fitness with garage-gym-minded people like yourself who would be willing to be that accountability partner and you can find us at EndofThreeFitness.com.

I share those common mistakes as a person who has made them and as result of surveying thousands of garage gym athletes at End of Three Fitness who say they have the exact same problems.

Saying "avoid those mistakes" is easier said than done. I know most people believe they can do it all themselves, and then get discouraged about their space or focus on the lack of equipment. No matter what I say. So I have solution for you.

Stop acting like you are an average Joe and start acting like an *Athlete*— your shift in perspective will be huge.

- An Athlete is serious about training.

- An Athlete follows real programming.

- An Athlete has accountability from their team and other athletes.

- An Athlete has standards they follow and strive for.

- An Athlete gets it done, knows things aren't always fair, and still keeps moving!

- An Athlete starts and sticks.

Pity parties aren't fun, and excuses are useless. If you want to see success in your garage gym the solution is simple. Start acting like an athlete and quit treating yourself as an average human being. Start and Stick!

Now, I feel like we have garage gyms covered from the shoulders up, so now let's jump into some of the more technical stuff.

Chapter 4

Ammunition: Helping Others See the Light

Do you want to work out in your underwear and save $15,000 in the process?

I have worked out at home in my underwear once before . . . ok, maybe twice . . . alright, alright, maybe it was a few times. Still not sure if I am proud of that, but nonetheless, it has happened.

Now, I know building a garage gym is not the easiest thing to do, and often times it may have nothing to do with money or equipment. The biggest challenge can be a spouse, roommate, parent, etc.

This chapter exists just for that reason. In this chapter we justify to your spouse, parents, or whoever; that spending money on a garage gym is worth it. It may even help you if you need a little extra convincing. It can be an uphill battle, but you have to take the approach that it is like investing; spend money to make money.

First, you have to know I am about to drop a sizable amount of information on you, but stick with me! We are going to start with some dollar signs, percents, and a little math. Don't worry; I do the math for you.

Unfortunately, there are not large studies done on the return on investment (ROI) for garage gymers or home-gym exercisers (I know, weird, right?). *But* there are a ton of studies on the ROI for corporate wellness programs instituted at large companies. I'll save you the headache of reading all that junk, because I did, and here's the average I came up with after reading way too many pages:

- The average ROI for every $1 spent was $3 to $5; and $1 to $13 in extreme outliers.

To explain: A company spends $1 on your health by providing a gym or wellness program and you garner them $3 to $5 by being more productive, not taking sick days, etc.

Furthermore, in other studies, a simple health and fitness program can generate

- An out-of-pocket health insurance savings of 27 percent.

I'm thinking of a cool tagline . . . 27 reps could save you 27 percent on health insurance, or more. Now all I need is a computer-animated gecko to make it stick. That principle is pretty simple. If you are fit and healthy you can lower your health insurance costs by 27 percent.

Alright, you got those numbers? Let's take it to the garage gym—breaking down that info into a family situation. Healthcare is too crazy and ever changing to give you a perfect example, so let me give a general example and you estimate from there.

If a family of four has an average out-of-pocket spending in health care of $5,000 annually—meaning they maxed out an annual deductible, *not* just monthly premiums—with small things like prescriptions, perhaps a minor surgery, checkups . . . *Boom* . . . maxed out at $5,000.

- Using that example if you were to implement operation garage gym (get healthy): $5,000 deductible at 27 percent savings = $1,350

Next, you have a current gym membership—most likely one you are going to get out of to pursue a garage gym. Keeping with our example, for a family membership you may be averaging $200/month and that is conservative considering some northeastern CrossFit® gyms charge $200/month per person.

- No gym membership: $15/ month - $200/ month = $180–$2400/year

I put the $15/month in there for those who pursue something like Planet Fitness. But to be honest, if Planet Fitness is your cup of tea, a garage gym most likely will not work for you.

I know the numbers are getting pretty deep, but just one more thing. Let's say you make the purchase of a complete garage gym for around $2,500 (higher end). Assuming you use it regularly, your health should increase and you should be more productive and free up more time to earn more money. Considering the corporate wellness studies, we will take an average and say for every $1 you spend on your garage gym, you will get $5 back in your earning potential.

– ROI from garage gym purchase of $2,500 = $12,500

BOOM!

The next time you are getting hassled for wanting to buy expensive garage gym equipment or to do a DIY project, just try the ole every-dollar-I-spend-will-come-back-5-fold argument. Works every time! Ok, maybe not every time.

The grand total there would be $16,250 (so I actually rounded down from $15,000) you just saved by deciding to work out at home! That's hard to believe and definitely in no way scientific, and it is completely dependent on your personal situation. I know some of those savings may overlap—time in the gym is time away from work, etc.

BOTTOM LINE: Being healthy saves you money!

And we aren't done.

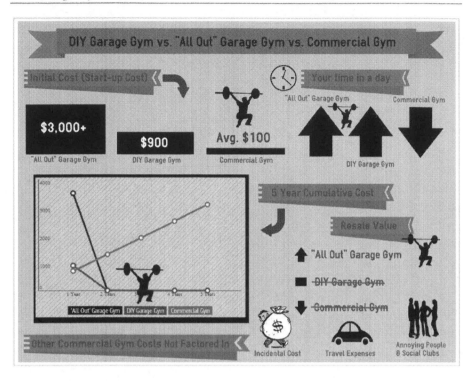

In an attempt to make this the most comprehensive book ever written on garage gyms, I have to go one step further in weighing the options of garage gyms vs. commercial gyms. Not only that, I would like to compare expensive garage gyms, DIY garage gyms, and commercial gyms.

Let's compare an "All Out" garage gym, a DIY garage gym, and a commercial gym.

Defining the gyms . . .

- "All Out" Garage Gym: The Garage Gym Athlete who really has no limit with the budget and would prefer to purchase everything. However, we are not talking about a rich-guy garage gym; all estimates are still feasible and on the low end.

- DIY Garage Gym: For the athlete on a budget who prefers to build, unless it is not feasible; i.e. no DIY barbells or plates, but everything else is fair game. You learn how to build *everything*.

- Commercial Gym: The globo gym! Your big-timers like LA Fitness and Life Time Fitness.

First, we will look at startup costs.

- "All Out" Garage Gym: A solid equipment package from a high-quality manufacturer will come in at just over $3,000.

- DIY Garage Gym: I created my first garage gym for $871, but with all the new knowledge updated in these pages you will be able to do it for $500, or less.

- Commercial Gym: Generally, if no specials are running, you will end up paying a signup fee and your first monthly dues. This leaves you, on average, at about $100.

Winner in startup costs goes to the commercial gym. Next, we have a big one; your time.

Time Considerations

- "All Out" Garage Gym & DIY Garage Gym: After the initial costs, a lot of the considerations for these two are exactly the same. With a garage gym, your time is going to increase. You don't need to muster up the energy to get up extremely early or in the evening, and scrounge together all the items you "need" for the gym. Wake up, roll into the garage, and get fit! *Note: If you want to get really technical, factor in the DIY time.*

- Commercial Gym: Commercial gyms are a time suck! You have the commute (5 to 20+ minutes), the check-in-put-my-stuff-away-and-get-to-the-exercise-equipment dance (10 minutes), the waiting-on-randoms-doing-the-exercise-incorrectly show-down (10 minutes), the hi-I-see-my-neighbor conversation (5 minutes). Do some of that in reverse and we are at over an hour—without factoring in the workout!

Overall the winner, by a landslide, will be the garage gym.

But what about in the long run?

Five-Year Cumulative Costs

I am not getting into a huge debate on how to break down the costs here. I went through accounting and finance in college so I know there are more business-appropriate ways to look at this, but that's not what we are doing. We are going to look at it very simply. How much did it cost me this year? The next year, ask yourself the same question, and so on and so forth.

- "All Out" Garage Gym: You have the expensive first year, and then you should really never have to factor in any other costs, especially if it is high-quality equipment.

- DIY Garage Gym: Same as the "All Out" Garage Gym, year one holds all the costs, and then it's smooth sailing. Considering it is DIY, and depending on your craftsmanship, your DIY garage gym equipment may have a 5 to 10 year shelf life. All of my DIY equipment has made it past the 5-year mark easily.

- Commercial Gym: This just keeps going up and up. It is basically the buy or lease argument. A lease has you pouring money into a service, more or less, with no ownership. You keep shelling out money and your ROI is your health.

That means in the 5-year timeline the DIY garage gym will be the winner.

Resale Value

This is a minor factor, but it is worth a mention.

- "All Out" Garage Gym: You will be able to recoup some of your initial costs by reselling your "All Out" Garage Gym equipment.

- DIY Garage Gym: Even if you are an awesome carpenter, you could only sell your DIY equipment for a few bucks on craigslist, at best. You may have to actually pay someone to haul it off.

- Commercial Gym: Absolutely no resale value.

This gives the All Out garage gym the advantage in resale value.

Other Considerations

"All Out" Garage Gym: Safety. Installation mistakes. Shipping time/costs.

DIY Garage Gym: Safety. DIY mistakes.

Commercial Gym: Travel expenses—commuting adds up. The globo gyms can suck you in with their $9 eggs and $7 protein shake smoothies that you know you will fall prey to at least a few times. People are always a factor in a commercial gym (not garage gym) setting and you need to decide if you like the people, or not.

In the end, you have to decide what works best for you.

Chapter 5

The Preamble: Canceling Gym Contracts and Saving Money

Now, some of you don't have a gym membership or a garage gym, which means you can just start from scratch. Lucky you! For those of you with a gym membership—what are you going to do?

Honestly, if you are at a major globo gym it will be tough. They have near ironclad contracts with a sea of lawyers behind them. It will be an uphill battle, but that doesn't mean it is not worth a try!

Getting out of a Gym Contract

- First, check your contract and see exactly what it says (keep this in mind for my fourth point)!

- Second, talk to a salesperson or client manager at the gym *while keeping your cool* about getting out of the contract early, and your options for doing so.

- Third, is it a year or more contract? If so, some states have laws that assert if you are in a contract of 1 to 2 years you can get out of it with written 30-day's notice.

- Fourth, what did they promise in the contract? Is there a service in the contract they have not been doing? Finding a discrepancy could help you get out!

- Fifth, are you moving or have you recently lost/changed your job? Sometimes if you reasonably explain a legitimate situation you are in, they may actually be cool about it.

If none of that works . . .

- Can someone take over your membership? A lot of gyms allow this.

- Will it be more cost effective to cancel and pay a termination fee or tell them you want to cancel and pay the remainder of the monthly payments?

- Are you able to successfully fake your own death? Okay, I'm kidding about this one.

Lastly, whether you are leaving a big or small gym, don't look back! Welcome to the start of fitness freedom.

You're one step closer to working out in your underwear!

Once you are out of your dysfunctional gym relationship you can start the other prep-work.

There will be a transition time for most where you may not have a gym. During this time you will need to save money for your garage gym and move your body, also known as bodyweight workouts and we have some listed in the bonus chapters of this book.

Garage gyms can be expensive, but they don't have to be.

This is what my first garage gym came out to be:

- Barbell, Plates, Kettlebells, and Clamps = $600

- Initial DIY Projects = $241

- Miscellaneous = $30

- Total = $871

For $871, I now have:

- (1) - 45 lb. Olympic Bar

- (3) - Kettlebells (35 lb., 55 lb., and 70 lb.)

- (2) - 45 lb. bumper plates

- (2) - 35 lb. bumper plates

- (2) - 25 lb. bumper plates
- (2) - 10 lb. bumper plates
- (2) - 5 lb. plates
- A power rack with pull-up bar
- Parallettes
- Weight rack storage
- Rings
- Plyometric box
- Medicine ball
- Tire for dragging and odd object lifting
- Squat/Press stands
- Bench press stands
- Bench
- Reverse hyper
- Speed rope

The funny thing is I didn't even go the cheapest route. If you are in the same boat I was, here are some tips for scrounging up some money for that garage gym.

Quick Tips for Saving Money

– Create a budget. Too easy, right? All of your money *will* go somewhere; be in control of that direction. Determine how much your garage gym will cost and how much you can save each month towards that goal.

– Get out of debt. This is a big one. My wife and I barely had any consumer debt when we got married, it was pretty much student loans that were killing us. Even if you only eliminate one small debt or a credit card, that is extra money in your pocket every month.

Now, if it is going to take a little while to save up for a garage gym, here is my challenge to you. Save at least $50 (eat out two times less this month) to build the plyometric box, the DIY kettlebell, and lastly, the quick and easy DIY pull-up bar. All of those projects are listed in the DIY portion of this book. Next, use a combination of that equipment and the body-weight program provided in this book. Those two actions should get you in great shape and keep you busy while you are gym-less and saving up the needed cash.

Don't start working out in your underwear yet—you're not ready. The underwear is an earned privilege!

BOTTOM LINE: Take control of your money, save for a gym, and focus on workouts you can do RIGHT NOW.

Alright, are you ready for a garage gym?

Chapter 6

Your First Step: The Big Purchase

It is time to start taking the steps to having your very own garage gym. Let's get started!

Step 1: The big purchase

The big purchase has to be the first thing you do when you are starting a serious garage gym. It means you are fully committed and the big purchase will help keep you accountable. This is the stuff you cannot build yourself or may be too challenging to find used; i.e. barbells, plates, kettlebells, etc.

Another reason to do the big purchase first is because it can take up to two weeks for the order to come in, depending on the company you use. This will give us time to set up shop in the garage and get ready for some serious training once the equipment is delivered. First, you have to decide what you need.

- Do you want or need rubberized bumper plates?

- Do you want only iron plates?

- Do you care if you have new or used equipment?

I didn't go the least expensive route when I first started my garage gym. I bought it all new and I bought the colored, rubberized bumper plates (expensive). If you buy plain black or go the used route you can get it all for much cheaper than I did. You don't need *all* bumper plates for a garage, and we will cover more on this in the barbell buyer's guide bonus chapter. Now, let's make the big purchase. You have four options:

1. Craigslist

Craigslist is full of people who thought they may enjoy a garage gym at one point in their life, but now their equipment is just junk that clutters their garage (don't be that guy!). The deals you can find on craigslist are insane, people selling thousands of dollars worth of weights for pennies on the dollar. It's crazy, and good for you and me. If you live in a big city, or near a big city, you will have a ton of good deals. The only thing I have found is that bumper plates are not easy to come by these days. I think the type of people who buy bumper plates are relatively serious about working out and are less likely to get rid of them. If you find anyone selling bumper plates below industry average, *don't hesitate!* I have found that some people sell their weight sets cheap and almost treat you like a trash haul away service. I made the mistake of not taking a great deal because I didn't want a lot of this guy's "other crap," but he wouldn't sell any of it individually. If it is a good deal, be the trash service, and throw other stuff away and keep what you came for.

Tips for craigslist

- Don't get murdered (be safe)

- Always negotiate (low ball 'em)

- Be patient

If you are going to go the craigslist route, be sure to read my bonus chapter on how to automate your garage gym shopping, which will make this a breeze. Next, you can go traditional and shop in store.

2. In store

There are two stores that you can go check out, or you can even order from them online: Academy and Dick's Sporting Goods.

I mention these options mainly for the plates. They have good package deals that come with a lot of iron plates and a barbell, and it is very affordable.

However, I recommend even if you get one of these package deals only use the barbell as your "extra," as the barbells they have are low quality.

I think you should order a good barbell using the guidelines set out for you in the "Barbell Buyer's Guide" chapter, and not rely on one from an in-store purchase. A barbell is the nucleus for the garage gym; you don't want it to be a piece of crap.

Back to online shopping. What can't you get on Amazon?

3. Amazon

Amazon has a lot of good deals, but they are not always available. I like to shop around for sets of bumper plates. I have found that to buy individual plates on Amazon is just like buying anywhere else.

However, they do have a lot of good deals on sets of bumper plates. Also their bars are pretty affordable, but as I said, you want a great barbell. The key here is that you are looking for anything with free shipping.

4. The big boys: equipment retailers

There are a few equipment retailers out there which have extremely high-quality products, and some even made in the USA.

To buy all of your equipment at these places would be a little pricy, but certainly worth it with their guarantees and quality products.

If you can afford it, go for it. If you cannot afford it, I would recommend at least getting your barbell from one of these places. They have a wide variety of barbells to choose from.

But there is a strategy to shopping with these vendors. To learn my recommendations on shopping for their equipment please visit:

– www.EndofThreeFitness.com/equipment

Hopefully I have pointed you in a good direction. Now order your weight, package, barbell, or whatever it is today so we can move on and start your second step.

Seriously. Go make your big purchase, then come back to this book and move to Step 2.

Chapter 7

Your Second Step: Getting Ready

You have to embrace the idea of street parking! Meaning, yes, the car may no longer fit in the garage. It's okay.

When it comes to garage gyms, there are two options.

- Option one: you can have a garage with a gym in it, or . . .
- Option two: you can have a gym that is in the shell of a garage.

In other words, you can either maintain a garage for storage and all your household items, or you can fully dedicate your garage to being a gym and nothing else. The more viable option for most will be option one. Either way you are probably going to have to declutter. Organization and storage are your two priorities at this point.

Storage Ideas

If you are not an organized person, it is time to change—if you want a garage gym, that is. If you have a lot of stuff that you need to keep (yes, getting rid of stuff is a real option), you will have to get creative. Quick suggestions:

- Hang storage containers from the ceiling
- Have a dedicated wall for stackable containers
- Move things to a storage unit (not ideal, due to the monthly cost that you're trying to save by doing this in the first place)
- Throw things away
- Garage sale

If you have a lot of stuff in your garage that you would not mind getting rid of, have a garage sale. This does two things for you, obviously: The first thing is it gives you room for a garage gym. The second awesome thing a garage sale can do for you is it may completely pay for your equipment! Now you really have no excuse.

Bottom line: You don't need a ton of space, but you will need a dedicated portion of the garage for lifting weights.

Clean up, clean out, and keep it clean.

You will have to get creative and organized. I recommend having one side of the space for "garage" items, and one side for gym items. However you do it, just make sure there is enough space for you to work out, which requires a little planning.

Luckily, the planning for this gym is as easy as reading through all the DIY projects we are planning to build in the next section of this book.

Make sure you have enough space for the projects you want to build. You can cherry-pick which projects you like and do not like. Once you have made up your mind you can sketch it on paper, draw it on a whiteboard, or even tape it out on your garage floor.

The more realistic you can picture it, the better off you will be. This way we do not work ourselves into a corner here. Do not skip planning — make sure you have a good idea of where absolutely everything will go.

Oh, and if you are married, like me, be sure to run all this stuff by your wife or husband. Maybe that should have been step one . . . *oops*.

After the garage is empty and you have a plan, it would be a great idea to get your flooring situated before any equipment arrives.

You do not need to completely redo your garage gym with a specific type of flooring. All you need is enough to where your weights would hit the rubber and not the concrete, or just enough for you to stand on. Buying it one piece at a time is perfectly fine. Flooring will make lifting safer and it will protect your garage floor and your weights. Both of which we do not want damaged.

And more importantly, it will absorb the shock when doing dead lifts. Take it from me, after doing thousands of dead lifts on concrete and paying the price in my neck, I now deadlift on rubberized flooring only.

Here are your options for flooring:

Once upon a time, I recommended getting flooring at Home Depot, Lowes, sporting goods stores, or even Amazon. However, I have found that the flooring from these places can be a bit too soft, which matters if you are going to lift heavy weight.

You best best is Tractor Supply Co.

This option really only works if you have a Tractor Supply Co. in your local area, but a lot of people do. You can check out their website www.tractorsupply.com and type in your zip code to find a store near you. You are looking for horse stall mats. They aren't super cheap, but you only need one or two pieces to use as your lifting platform.

You can explore further options, but these mats are typically very heavy and will kill you on shipping if you order online. If you find free shipping online, do it.

Alright!

Are you ready to build!?

Chapter 8

Your Third Step: DIY or Decide

Everything you have ever wanted to achieve in fitness can be done in your garage; we are firm believers of this. However, it will take dedication on your part. If you want to join the garage gym revolution you have two options, in my opinion.

- YOU CAN BUILD IT

- YOU CAN BUY IT

Now, the next part of this book will lay out numerous DIY projects. But in this chapter, I will highlight the items I recommend building. You certainly have the option of just buying everything for your gym. To really make it yours, however, and to save some cash, you can build a few pieces of your own. I recommend, building these four projects to start:

- Plyometric Box

- Power Rack

- Medicine Ball

- Parallettes

These first few items will help you get started with a core garage gym, and you could get it all done in one dedicated weekend.

Plyometric Box

- The first project is a plyometric box. One sheet of plywood, six cuts to suit the size you need, some glue, screws, and you are done! A plyometric box can be used for box jumps, dips, step-ups, box squats, and any other creative exercise you can think of. It is a very quick and easy project. It will only cost about $20, take you about 30 minutes, and is not very difficult to complete.

Power Rack

- The second project is a little more difficult and time consuming: a power rack. However, if you build this project, and take care of it, it will last a long time. It will also give you a great training capability. You will be able to squat with safety bars and make use of a pull-up bar. You can make any modification you like to suit your needs. If this project is too advanced for you, I recommend some cement buckets and 4x4s (also listed in this book).

Medicine Ball

- The third project is very quick and easy: a medicine ball. Just cut open a basketball, fill it with pool salt (not sand) and patch it up. Now you have a medicine ball! A medicine ball is great for wall ball shots (squatting with and throwing to a target 10 feet away), weighted sit-ups, medicine ball cleans, and many other exercises. It is a must when starting a garage gym.

Parallettes

- The fourth project is also quick and easy: parallettes. Parallettes are great for deficit push-ups, L-sits, dips, pass-throughs, and many other exercises. This project just takes a few cuts of PVC, some PVC cement, and you are good to go. Very easy and a great addition to a garage gym.

These projects are just the start, but with a solid foundation and these few items, you will have enough equipment to have a very simple and effective garage gym.

As you become more experienced and learn more about how you operate in a garage gym you can slowly expand your DIY arsenal or purchase the additional items you need.

As with any do-it-yourself project, unfamiliarity with the tools and process can be dangerous. If you are at all uncomfortable or inexperienced working on DIY projects (especially projects involving dangerous tools), please reconsider doing the job yourself. It is very possible on any DIY to damage your property, create a hazardous condition, or harm yourself or others.

Be careful!

Section Two

The Simple Life: DIY Projects

Chapter 9

Do it Yourself—Do it Safely

This section of the book—The Simple Life: DIY Projects—does not read like a traditional book. As I am not telling a story, but rather, providing you with a reference guide on how I built my very first garage gym with these DIY projects.

There are better ways, safer ways, and overall many different ways to assemble a garage gym. This is simply an account of how I did it.

Projects in this book should be viewed as entertainment only. End of Three Fitness and the creators, will not be held responsible for any injury due to the misuse or misunderstanding of any DIY project or the misunderstanding of what this section of the book was designed for.

If you like these DIY projects and want to see more than what is contained in this book, and to see updated versions of these projects, or for a full list of DIY projects, please visit the following site:

- www.EndofThreeFitness.com/DIY

Before we start the DIY section, we must start with the laws and rules of the garage gym:

Garage Gym Laws

1. A Garage Gym Athlete may not allow a human being to become injured or, through a sedentary lifestyle, allow a human being to come to harm.

2. A Garage Gym Athlete must do everything in his/her power to become a complete badass, except where such efforts would conflict with the first law.

3. A Garage Gym Athlete must protect the existence of the garage gym at all costs as long as such protection does not conflict with the first or second laws.

Garage Gym Rules

1. Clean It: I must admit that I come to fault on this one. You are now the "gym owner." Pick up your weights, sweep the floors, and don't let it look trashy.

2. Equipment Checks: I recommend equipment checks every six weeks, especially if you have a lot of DIY equipment. You need to make sure your equipment is safe and ready for use. Every six weeks I like to check that all bolts are tightened and that there are no loose screws. Also, check that your equipment is not rusting and make sure it is protected from the elements.

3. Avoid Precarious Situations: I developed this rule after I found myself under 285 pounds held by one screw on top of my plyometric box, ready to do floor press. I realized that if I failed to unrack the weight properly or if that screw gave out, I would most likely end up with a crushed skull. Be safe and don't put yourself in any questionable situations with a lot of weight and crappy rigs.

4. Invite Friends, but Don't Charge Them: Invite your friends to work out in your garage gym, but never try to get their money. Unless you don't want friends anymore. Having a garage gym and starting a CrossFit® Box are totally different. Decide what you want to do.

5. Hold Yourself Accountable: You are going to need something or someone to help you train. You will also need to track your progress.

6. No One Rep Maxes Alone: Don't do it! Working out with a barbell alone is kind of like flying an airplane; 99.9 percent of the time you are going to be just fine, but if you encounter that .1 percent, the result will be catastrophic. Don't put yourself in a situation where you are more likely to find the .1 percent.

7. Learn to Be a Minimalist: While you should not break the "Avoid Precarious Situations" rule you need to learn that you do not need a lot of equipment to be successful in a garage gym. For almost six months all I had was a barbell and some weight and I still managed to become pretty fit. I then decided to expand a little, but only because I wanted to. You don't need fancy equipment or the latest shoe to be good at what you do.

8. Become an Expert: This is a personal rule but it may help you too. Become an expert; learn, read, and grow. You have to know what to do to make yourself better. If you even want to think about inviting someone to your garage gym to work out you should know what you are talking about. Always know the *why* about everything that interests you.

Alright, aspiring Garage Gym Athlete. I think you are ready for the projects.

Let's begin!

Chapter 10

How to Build a Plyometric Box

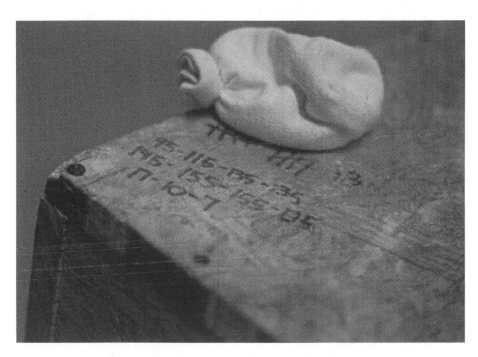

What You Need to Know

- **Cost:** Around $20

- **Time:** 30 minutes

- **Difficulty:** Medium

This is one of the easiest and most important DIY builds. The plyometric box will serve a lot of different purposes in your garage gym. When using a plyometric box be sure to do box jumps correctly; jump, land, full hip extension, and land or step down.

In this project you get a three-in-one box since it is a rectangular prism. Building a rectangular prism will give you three different sides to jump on which will be three different heights. This is great for different workouts and overall functionality.

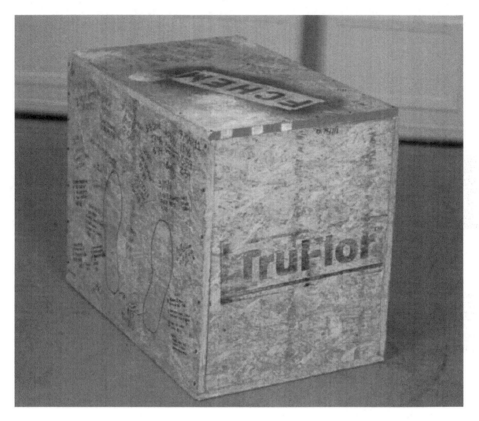

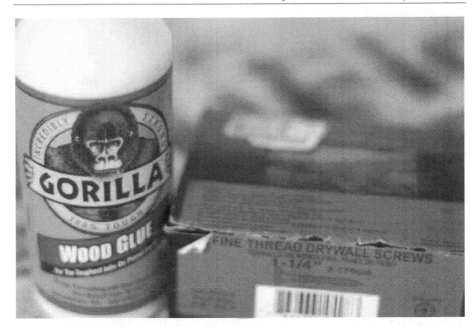

Materials Needed

- (1) - Piece of plywood (I got the cheap plywood generally used for flooring because it is tough. Get any plywood you want, so long as it is ¾ inch x 4 feet by 8 feet)

- (1) - Box of screws

- (1) - Bottle of Gorilla Wood Glue

Now, answer this question:

What kind of box do *you* want/need? Typical dimensions (and the ones used for this project):

- L = 30″

- W = 20″

- H = 24″

After mine was constructed I wish I had made the length 40″ since I like to do really high box jumps. You need to determine what you can handle and what you want. You can make it as tall or as short as you desire.

Step 1: Let's start cutting

You will need the following dimensions cut

- Two cuts at 30"x 22½"

- Two cuts at 30"x 20"

Trickiest part of the project

- 2x 18½"x 22½"(this cut will be the sides and will fit within the other pieces to make a streamline box)

Step 2: Gluing and screwing—what all DIY projects need

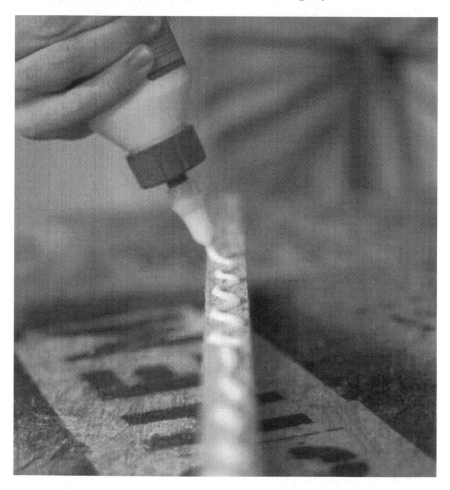

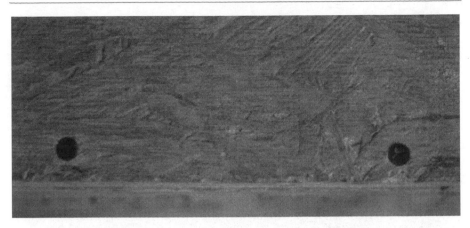

Now that you have all your pieces, simply put them together. (Refer to the picture of the box above—it is pretty self-explanatory.)

Anywhere wood will be touching wood, put a thin line of Gorilla Wood Glue.

I recommend starting with the base and two sides all touching. This will give it immediate stability and you can let it dry as needed.

While putting it together, I would put a screw spaced every 2 to 3 inches around the entire box. I tend to overkill things when building, but hey, if it falls apart you can only blame yourself, so make it *sturdy*. Mine has withstood a lot of jumping and I have even used it as an apparatus for floor press with nearly 300 pounds resting on it.

Easy! Get this one done!

Chapter 11

Build Your Own Power Rack

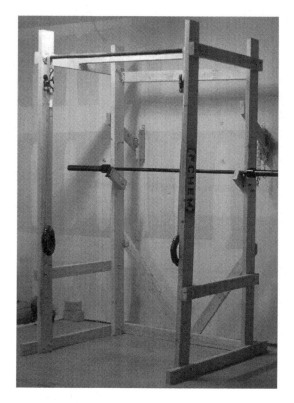

What You Need to Know

- **Cost:** Less than $100

- **Time:** 2 to 3 hours

- **Difficulty:** Medium

Your equipment arsenal is not complete without a power rack.

I did a lot of research in buying/making a power rack. I found a lot of good designs for homemade, but I found a lot of them were overdone and too expensive. Same with buying a power rack—way overpriced. Here is how you build one:

Step 1: Buy the following supplies

- (7) - 8' 2x4s
- (4) - 8' 2x6s
- (1) - 43″ galvanized pipe
- (2) - flanges
- (28) - 5″–6″ bolts with washers
- (1) - box 3½″ wood screws
- (1) – box flat screws
- 90-degree flat bracket
- (1) - Wood pencil

Chances are you may have some of this stuff lying around. As you can see from the first picture the design is very simple.

Step 2: Make sure you bought all DIY power rack materials

This option is still *wayyyyy* cheaper than commercial alternatives.

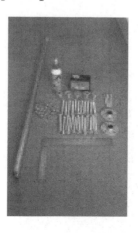

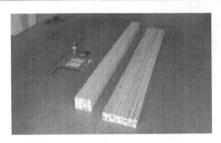

Step 3: Get to work (build your frames)

The rack can be scaled to the space you have available since the design is so simple. I kept mine simple with minimal cutting so it was a little bit bigger than it had to be. I did not want to mess with cutting pipe and having to rethread it so my frames were built around the pipe.

- First: Lay out your two 2x6s, and then cut your two 2x4s. What you are cutting is the upper support beam and the squat safety bar. Keep in mind if you have a low ceiling you want to make sure your face won't slam into it when doing pull-ups so keeping your 2x6s at 8 ft. is up to you. Also, since I made my squat safety bar permanent, you want to make sure that it is low enough for you to go all the way down on your squat without any problems.

    - I cut my top support beam and squat safety bar at 43 inches.

    - My top support beam is secured by two bolts drilled through on each end at 45- degree angles.

    - My squat beam is only secured by one bolt at each end.

- Second: Cut your bottom support beam. Mine extends well beyond each side of the rack. They were cut at 56 inches. The extra length adds support during normal and kipping pull-ups.

    - These too are secured by two bolts on each ends at 45-degree angles from one another.

    - At this point your frames should be built and you're almost done.

— Third: Your basic frame should be built. You may want to stand them up and see *exactly* where you want to place your flanges for the pull-up bar. I determined I wanted them pretty close to the top with just enough space for my chest to be above the bar and still have about 5 inches before my head would hit the ceiling.

　　— After you determine this, you can add your flanges. My suggestion is to secure a flange to one side, and then screw in the pipe. Next, screw the flange on the other side of the pipe and *then* secure it to your second frame. If you do it in any other order, you are adding unnecessary work.

A look at the frames:

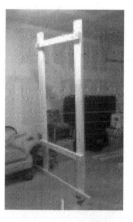

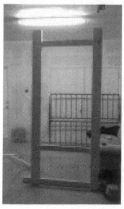

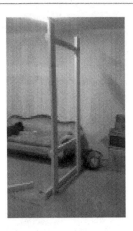

Step 4: Put the frames together

- Put the structure together on the ground starting with the pipe as stated above. After you have done this, you can add the back support beam as seen in the picture. It should be cut to whatever length measures between the two 56-inch bottom support beams.

- I know what you want to do now. You want to use it!

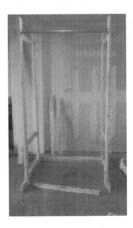

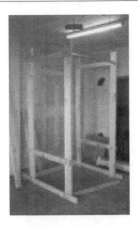

DO NOT do pull-ups on this structure yet. She's not ready.

At this point you should have your basic structure erected and all the basic framing done. All that is needed from here is a few extra support and brace beams for added structure support.

Step 5: Add support

All the cutting from here on is at your discretion. Here is what I added for more support.

- Two 45ish-degree braces running from the back support beam to the main vertical structure.

- Two top support beams. One mimics the bottom back support beam just at the top. The other was put in to connect the top of the structure from inside to inside.

- Next, I secured my structure to my wall studs. This means I can kip, swing, and go crazy without the structure moving.

- Last thing is to add your bar holders for squats. I cut mine about 10 inches and secured them with two bolts at 45-degree angles. Make sure they are tightened down really well.

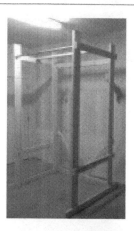

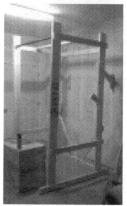

Without the use of glue, I simply secure my bolts once a month and make sure they are tight.

This rack should last a long time, and be the center piece of all your equipment; if something fails on it I would certainly take a Saturday to build a new one.

Chapter 12

DIY Wallball

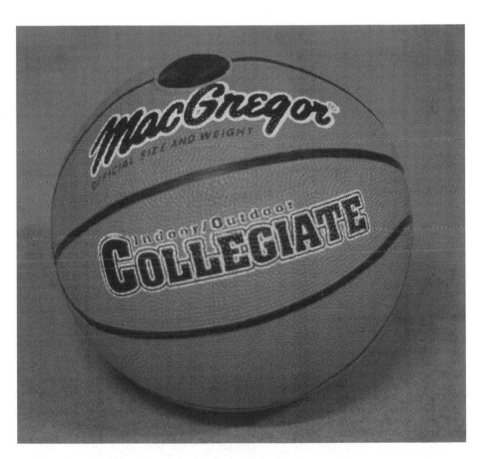

What You Need to Know

- **Cost:** $12

- **Time:** 20 minutes

- **Difficulty:** Easy

A project like this one makes it really hard for me to believe people do not have the time or money to work out at their home. This was a simple, affordable, and fun equipment build.

Materials Needed

- Rubber indoor/outdoor basketball
- Tire patch kit
- 40 pounds of salt pellets

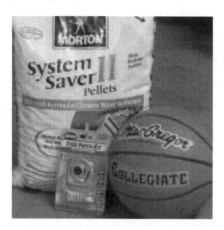

Step 1: Make incision

I started with an X-cut and then ended up making a square like shape where I could fit the bottle in the top.

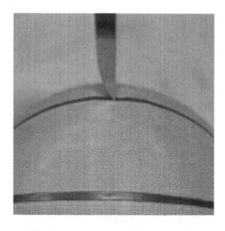

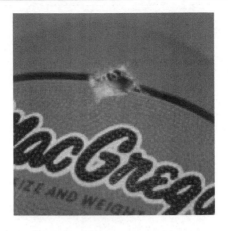

Step 2: Fill the ball with salt pellets

WHY SALT PELLETS? WHY NOT SAND?

- Salt pellets will NOT leak if you damage your ball after repeated use; sand will.

- Salt pellets will fully fill your basketball for better balance; sand will not.

- Salt pellets are just a little bit cheaper than sand.

- Salt pellets are easy to work with and to clean up.

I used the bottle for filling the ball 98 percent full. Then I had to shake it around to get that last pound of salt in there. I made mine a little over my goal of 20 pounds, but I left mine at around this weight because my scale kept fluctuating and I figured I'd rather be a little over than a little under—20 pounds would be optimal.

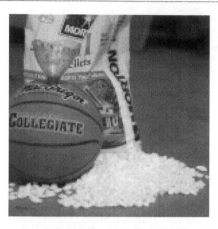

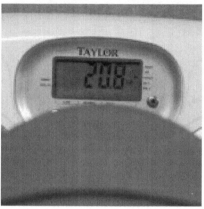

Step 3: This wall ball is no good with holes

Use the tire puncture kit—the largest size—and follow the directions to patch up your ball.

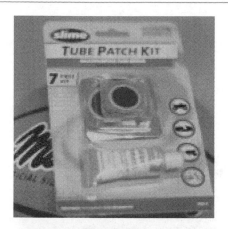

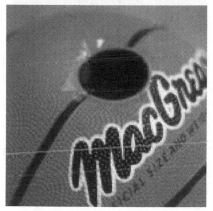

Chapter 13

How to Build Parallettes

What You Need to Know

- **Cost:** Less than $35

- **Time:** 30 minutes

- **Difficulty:** Easy

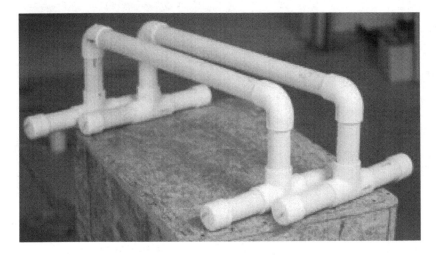

Parallettes are great for gymnastics workouts, or any workout for that matter, and are a great addition to your garage gym inventory! You can use them for handstand push-ups, push-ups, L-sits, and many other workouts.

Materials Needed

- (1) - 10′ x 1½″ PVC pipe
- (1) - Can PVC cement
- (4) - 1½″ 90-degree elbow joints
- (4) - 1½″ T-joints
- (8) - 1½″ PVC caps
- (1) - Piece of sandpaper (optional)

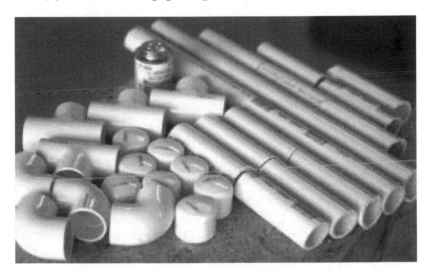

Now as you can see in the picture above, I already have my 10-foot PVC pipe cut down into pieces. The reason being is because I asked the guy at Home Depot if he would cut it for me, and he did! That is half the project right there. Whether you cut it or you get someone to cut it, here is what you will need.

- (12) - 6″ pieces
- (2) - 24″ pieces

As you can see that is a lot of cutting. Also, the guy didn't cut mine perfectly straight, but that is not a huge deal in this project. Now that you have everything, let's get to work.

To make sure everything fits properly you are going to have to take a pencil or piece of sand paper to clean all the edges of the cut PVC.

Another optional step is to rough the first inch of each piece of the PVC pipe. It helps the cement stick a little better, but it is not necessary.

Step 1: Clean up the edges

Everything should be cleaned up and ready for glue now.

Step 2: Main horizontal piece

The next thing we are going to do is build our main horizontal piece. All of this gluing and piecing together is pretty easy. The only thing you need to worry about is making sure you get everything straight. You can use a level if you want. I use the ground and my eye. For the main horizontal piece put some glue/PVC cement on the inside of the 90-degree elbow joint and on the outside of the horizontal piece. One side at a time!

Once you have both sides, lay the piece on the ground and make sure that both elbow joints are even, and that it will lay flat on the ground. Don't wait too long to do this. The cement gives you a very limited amount of time to adjust anything.

Step 3: Making the rest of the pieces

After you get these pieces you can go ahead and start making all the pieces you will need for the rest of the project.

- Glue caps onto 8, 6-inch pieces

- Glue 4, 6-inch pieces into the 90-degree T-joints

- Put the capped pieces inside of the T-joints

Here is the progression:

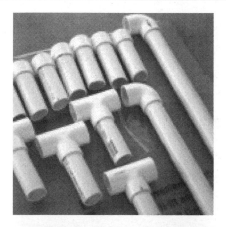

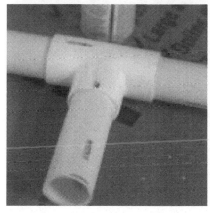

Everything to this point has been pretty easy, and it really doesn't get any harder, but if you are the guy who truly loves precision, then you are going to want to bust out your level. Like I said earlier, I just eyeball it, but that seems to bother a lot of people.

Step 4: Putting it all together

What we are going to do now is take the T-joint like in the picture and connect it to your main horizontal piece. If you screw this up, you just wasted a lot of time. Nobody wants wobbly or crooked parallettes. Here is what it looked like after I eyeballed it. I just used the ground to make sure it was straight and lined up the 6-inch piece with the 24-inch piece and made sure they looked right. Do this for all sides (4 total) and you should have yourself a nice pair of parallettes.

Good luck!

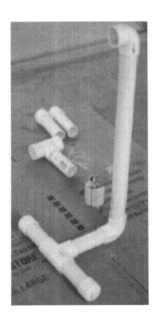

Chapter 14

How to Build a Slosh Pipe

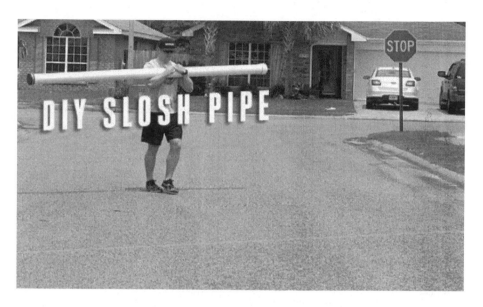

Have you ever heard of a slosh pipe? Well, let's talk about how to build a slosh pipe!

A slosh pipe is simply a PVC pipe filled 2/3, or less, with water. The term "slosh" is used because the water sloshes around inside the pipe, which makes this apparatus very challenging to move around.

The DIY slosh pipe comes in at one of the quickest, cheapest, and easiest DIY projects you can do; I highly recommend it—because you will get the biggest bang for your buck with a DIY slosh pipe.

This puppy has the ability to challenge every muscle in your body, and a lot of muscles you don't even know about, or rarely use. Personally, I am not a huge fan of traditional sit-ups and crunches for strengthening my core and prefer stabilization exercises to get the job done.

The slosh pipe will do just that, and much more. It can work on stabilization muscles in the core, your arms, back, chest, etc. Basically, you can use the slosh pipe for any exercise you can do with a barbell.

How to Build a Slosh Pipe

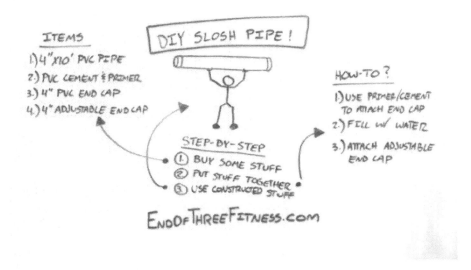

My amazing whiteboard artwork (above) breaks the entire project down to show how easy this project actually is, but there a few things I want to talk about.

What You Need to Know

- **Cost:** $25–$30

- **Time:** One hour (including time for PVC to dry)

- **Difficulty:** Easy

First, decide on what size you want. I built (and recommend) a PVC pipe that is 4 inches in diameter and 10 feet long. It makes it easy because you can buy that exact size and avoid any cutting.

Depending on *your* size and strength you could also do a 3-inch diameter pipe and vary lengths at 6 feet or 8 feet, etc. I know some people who go even wider in diameter—it really is up to you. I like the size I have, and it is very challenging to use. You can always add or take away water in the pipe to make it harder/easier to use. No matter the size, the instructions are the same.

Got your DIY slosh pipe materials?

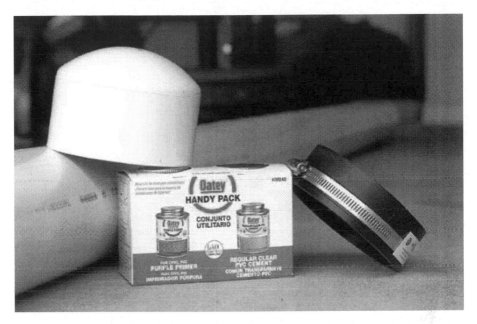

Materials Needed

- (1) - 4"x 10' PVC pipe
- (1) - 4"PVC end cap
- (1) - 4"rubber adjustable end cap
- (1) - PVC primer/cement combo pack
- Water

Step 1: Apply primer and cement

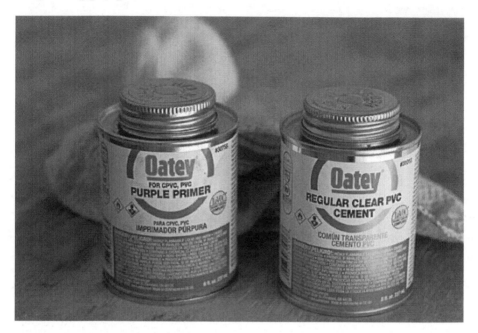

Nothing tricky here. Follow the instructions on the back of these two cans and you will be just fine.

Step 2: Seat the end cap

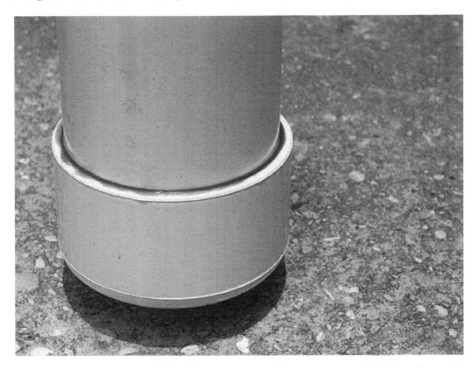

Make sure that you get the PVC all the way seated inside the cap. Standing the pipe straight up will provide enough pressure to make sure it is fully seated. Just watch out for any spillover from the PVC cement.

Make sure you let the PVC cement fully cure before you start to add water.

Step 3: Add water . . . the right amount

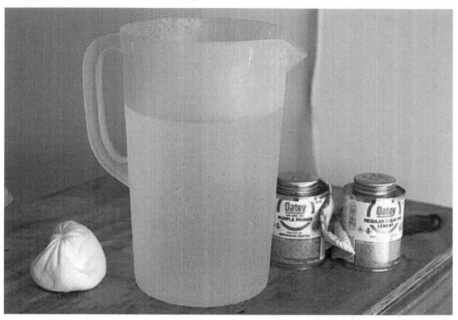

You waited long enough for the PVC cement to dry, right? Good.

Now, add water.

How much water should you add?

Keep in mind you only want this thing to weigh roughly 40 pounds. I added too much water at first and it was somewhere around the 55-pound mark and, let me tell you, a 55-pound slosh pipe danced me all around my front yard and up and down my street. I let some water out to get it to 40 pounds total weight.

Keep it simple. Just weigh how much your PVC materials are and then after that each gallon of water you add will be an additional 8.34 pounds. For my slosh pipe, that came out to around four gallons inside the pipe.

The weight of the pipe is significantly different if you made a 10-foot slosh pipe as opposed to an 8-foot pipe. Just play with it until you get it right. For me, a 10-foot, 4-inch-diameter slosh pipe weighing roughly 40 pounds is perfect—not too easy and not too tough. *Optional: add a few capfuls of bleach to make sure the water doesn't get gross.*

Step 4: Add the adjustable end cap

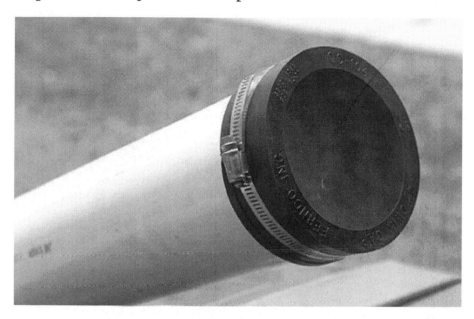

Make sure the rubber is seated and flush on the PVC then tighten it down. Next, it is time to use this thing!

DIY Slosh Pipe in Action

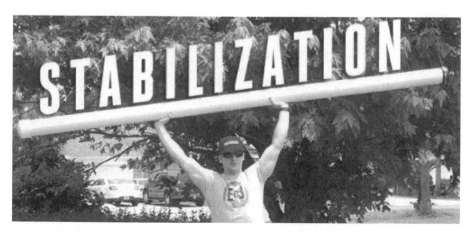

A slosh pipe is no walk in the park, especially if you are not accustomed to stabilization exercises, or if you put too much water in at first, like I did.

Core stabilization is *huge*! Being able to properly stabilize your core can aid in injury prevention, improve your balance, and even reduce blood lactate levels post workout to help you recover better and reduce soreness.

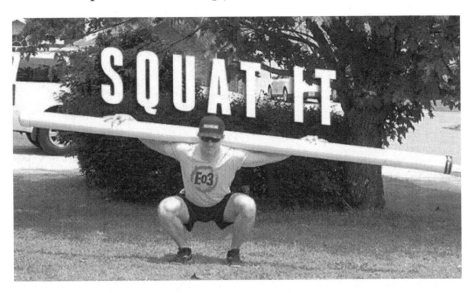

It really doesn't matter what you are doing with a slosh pipe—if you don't want to drop it, you will learn to stabilize every muscle in your body. Little tiny muscles will scream at you after first use, and really large muscles will be sore just from the confusion of all this.

You can do anything with a slosh pipe; you can bench press it, overhead press it, squat it, deadlift it, lunge with it, or just walk with it on your back. It's all good, but the number one thing I recommend is a Zercher walk.

The Zercher slosh pipe walk.

The picture at the beginning of this chapter is the Zercher walk. Cradle the slosh pipe in your arms and just talk a stroll down the street. Honestly, you will look a little like a drunk person when you first start, as you may stumble around quite a bit, but don't worry, it gets better.

Chapter 15

How to Build Jerk Boxes

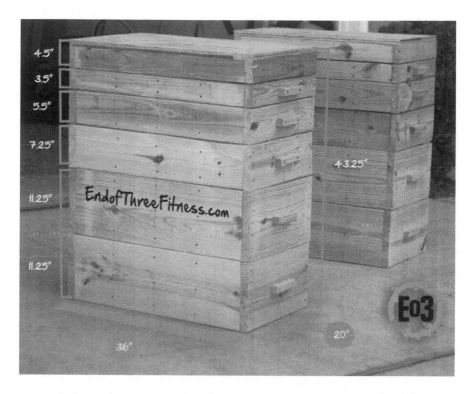

DIY jerk boxes—a project for the dedicated in training and DIY

What You Need to Know

- **Cost**: Around $200 (my exact cost was $236, but I bought too much wood)

- **Time**: Probably two weekend days—if working alone (I had a partner)

- **Difficulty**: Medium

Before we jump into how to build these hefty boxes, let's talk about a few things. First, what is a jerk box? After I finished this DIY project, one of my neighbors swung by my house and said, "What's that you built?" and I said they were jerk boxes.

She said, "Oh, so when someone is a jerk you put them in that box?"

Of course she was kidding, but by the same token, she didn't fully understand the point of jerk boxes. Let me briefly explain.

Jerk boxes serve two primary purposes:

- Jerk boxes give you the ability to lift at different heights and positions of a specific lift; for example, snatching from below the knee (and *many* other combinations)

- Jerk boxes also allow you to "jerk" heavy weight overhead and bring it back down to the boxes as opposed to the ground or your back. This allows for high-rep jerks and heavy jerks without having to re-rack or risk hitting your spine.

Obviously, dependent on your style of training, they can be quite useful. While that is the primary purposes of jerk boxes, I have been using them for a lot more, and you can too.

What I've been using jerk boxes for:

- Basically everything.

- Squats and presses.

- I have even used low boxes to act as my "safety bars" when going really heavy on squat.

- I have used them for heavy jerks.

- High box jumps.

- Dips.

- And more!

Jerk boxes are pretty awesome.

These things will take up quite a bit of space in your garage; you have been warned.

These boxes are sturdy. I thoroughly tested them at 285 pounds overhead and dropped many times on the boxes. I also did some lighter high-rep stuff to make sure the tops could take a beating. So far, the jerk boxes are holding up great.

Step 0 (preparation phase): End of Three Fitness DIY jerk boxes plus coffee

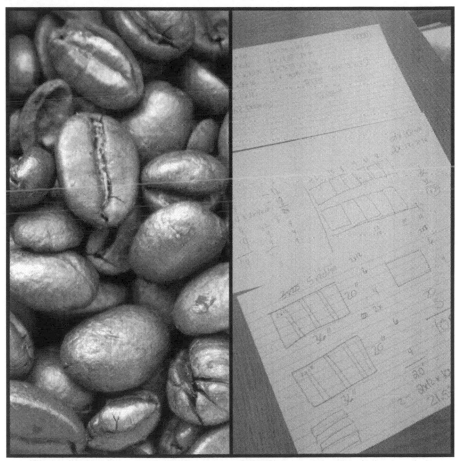

The jerk boxes consist of, in total, both stacks of boxes:

- All boxes are 36″x 20″—then heights are . . .

- 4 x 11¼"
- 2 x 7¼"
- 2 x 5½"
- 2 x 3½"
- 2 x 4½" Tops

This will put your boxes somewhere between 43¼ inches and 44 inches depending on how well they stack. Another thing to note is the 3½-inch box can be viewed as optional depending on how tall you are. If you are five feet eleven inches tall and above, build it. Below five feet eleven inches tall, it is optional.

Oh as for the "plus coffee," whatever source of artificial motivation you use--it may be time to load up on your favorite beverage; this is quite a project.

Step 1: Buy DIY jerk box material

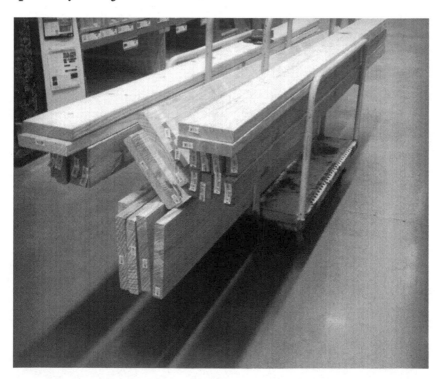

The previous picture is a little more wood than you will actually need. I experimented a little bit and tried to make it the strongest structure while using the least amount of wood—aka money.

Basically buy a crap ton of wood.

- (1) - Sheet of plywood, ½″
- (6) - 2 x 12 x 10
- (3) - 2 x 8 x 10
- (3) - 2 x 6 x 10
- (7) - 2 x 4 x 10
- (1) - 2 x 2 x 10
- (3) - 1 x 4 x 10
- (3) - Boxes 3″ drywall screws
- (1) - Box 1½″ drywall screws

Step 2: Start building your DIY jerk box frames

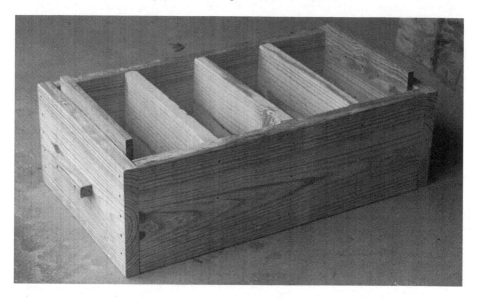

★★★I am only going to explain how to do this one time, as each frame/box measurement and construction will be the same, just using different wood size.★★★

To clarify, you will follow Steps 2 to 4 for all boxes; meaning all four of your 11¼-inch boxes, both of your 7¼-inch boxes, both of your 5½-inch boxes and both 3½-inch boxes. Step 5 explains how to build the tops.

Let's begin.

Make the following cuts on the 10-foot boards:

- Cut two 33-inch pieces
- Cut two 20-inch pieces

Those will basically be your frame pieces.

Put your 33-inch pieces and 20-inch pieces together using three to five (depending on board length—see main picture) 3-inch screws. The 33-inch pieces go on the inside of the 20-inch pieces, which will make for a perfect 36-inch x 20-inch frame.

Note: Since 3-inch screws can be hard to work with, all holes for this project were pre-drilled.

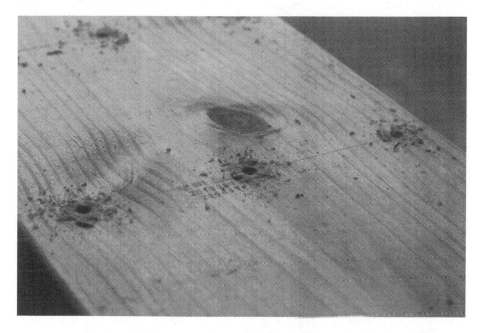

Now that you have your frame, you will need supports that will go on the inside of this frame.

Step 3: Inserting supports to your DIY jerk box frames

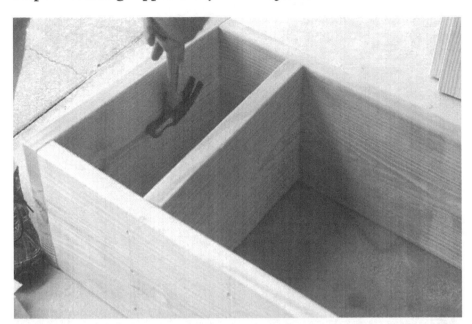

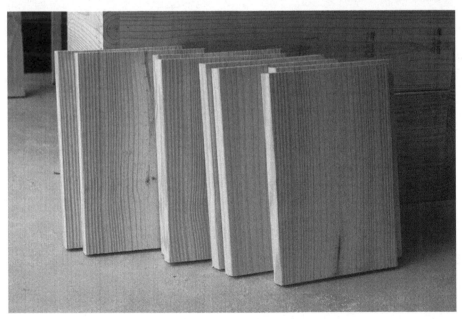

More cuts:

- Cut three 17-inch pieces (per box), which will be the inside supports

Wood is not perfect, so the inside pieces *should* all be 17 inches, but that is not always the case. You can easily measure, after you put your frame together, and if the inside of your frame is 16¾ inches, then cut three 16¾-inch pieces.

These inside support pieces will (and should be) a pretty tight fit, and a little wrangling may be in order; as seen in the hammer picture above.

The inside supports should be evenly spaced and placed:

- Measure a spot every 8¼ inches, which is where each of your 17-inch pieces will go.

- 3 screws for every support

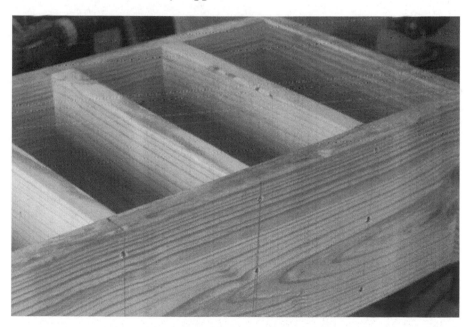

Step 4: Adding lips and handles to your DIY jerk boxes

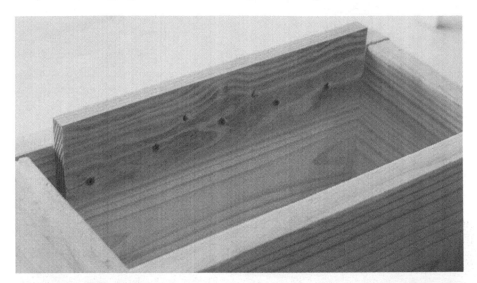

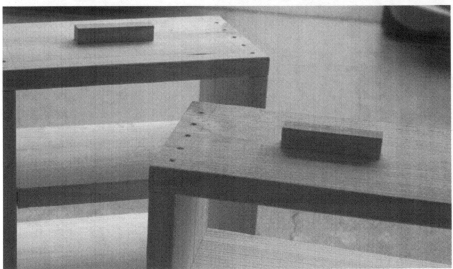

The "lips" will hold the boxes from sliding around when you drop the weight on top of it. There will be two lips per box, except for the tops.

LIPS: Cut and attach

- Cut two 15-inch lips for each box; using the 1 x 4 x 10 wood

- Attach with 5–7, 1½"screws

- **★★Make sure you alternate in a zigzag pattern like above (two screws). If you put all the screws in a straight line on the lip, it will move around too much.

HANDLES: Cut and attach

- Cut two 6-inch handles for each box; using 2 x 2 x 10 wood

- Attach with two 3-inch screws

- Measure to be in center of the box.

BONUS TIPS:

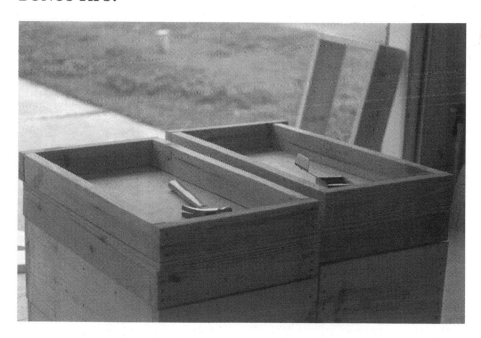

Here are a few tips that should help you while you are building boxes:

- Build frames on top of frames. As I stated earlier, wood is not perfect. If you build frames on top of other frames they will fit snuggly with very little gaps. If you build them on the perfectly level ground they will not fit as well.

- Pre-drill all holes

- Build one entire box—lips, handles and all—see how everything works; then you can pretty much start an assembly line process for the rest of your boxes. It gets a lot easier and faster after you fully understand how one box works.

Step 5: Building the tops to your jerk boxes

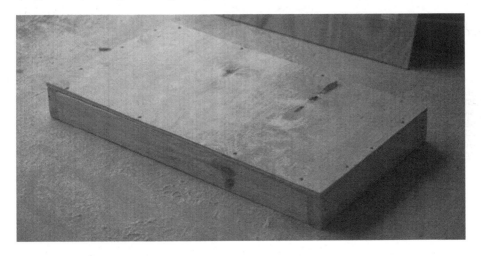

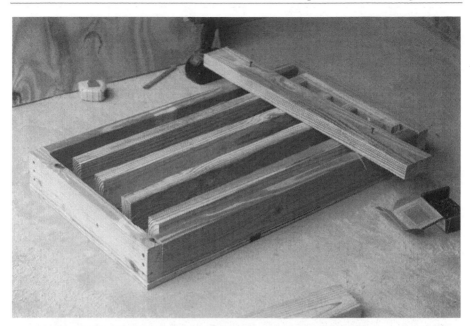

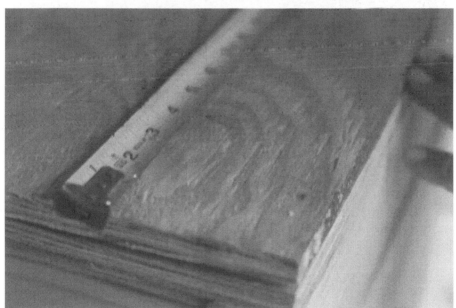

The End of Three Fitness DIY jerk box tops are double plywood, 2x4 supported tops. You will see a lot of jerk boxes with rubber padding on top to help lessen the amount of noise and to help absorb some of the impact. We decided to skip the rubber padding, as it is not necessary and will only add to your costs, but the choice is yours.

The top is made out of 2x4s and plywood.

For *one* top, you will need

- Two 33″ 2x4s
- Two 20″ 2x4s

Put those pieces together like the previous frames.

Cut plywood

- Two 36″ x 20″
- Attach one sheet of plywood to the top of the frame

Cut 2 x 4 supports (will go inside frame)

- Four 30″ 2x4s

The inside supports need to be evenly placed like in the picture above. There will also need to be a 1½-inch gap on each short side of the tops. This will make the "lips" from the other boxes fit easily to the tops.

Complicated part of project: Put on your thinking caps!

Now, you will need to evenly add the four 30-inch pieces. What we did was evenly place all the 2x4s. We then took an extra 2x4 and lightly drilled it in the box to hold all four pieces in place (shown in picture above). After that, just stand the box up and drill 1½-inch screws through the first sheet of plywood into the 2x4s. Your structure is almost complete. After all 30-inch 2x4s are secure, add the second sheet of 36-inch x 20-inch plywood to the top of the other piece of plywood.

You now have a completed top.

Now, build another one.

That's about it for this project. It is a lot of cutting and screwing, but fairly simple.

Completed Stack

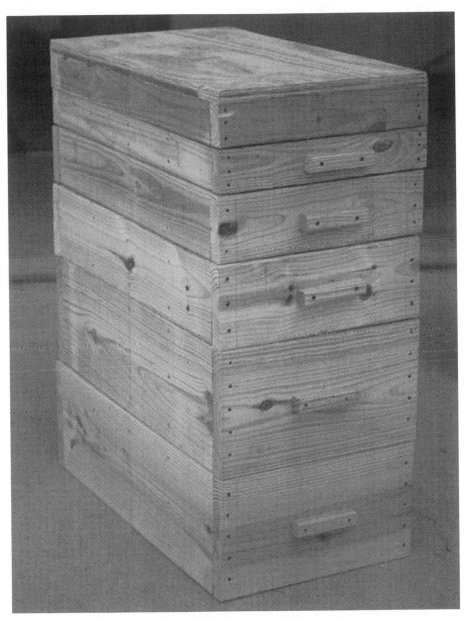

Other Considerations & Possible Issues:

- I did not add wood stops to the top of my boxes. My boxes are pretty level, and the weight doesn't roll off the box when I place it on top. However, for safety reasons or if your garage has a slight grade, screw some pieces on the top—both front and back—and that problem will be taken care of.

- I thought this would be a problem because I have heard of others having this problem. Some people say their jerk boxes "bounce all over the place" when they slam heavy weights on top of them. I am not having that problem at all. Our "lips" keep the boxes from moving front to back, but I haven't even really had side to side problems. If your boxes do not end up as level as you would have liked and they do bounce side to side, just add more lips to the sides as you did to the front and back. Problem solved, if it is a problem at all.

Good luck in building your jerk boxes!

Chapter 16

How to Make a DIY Prowler Sled

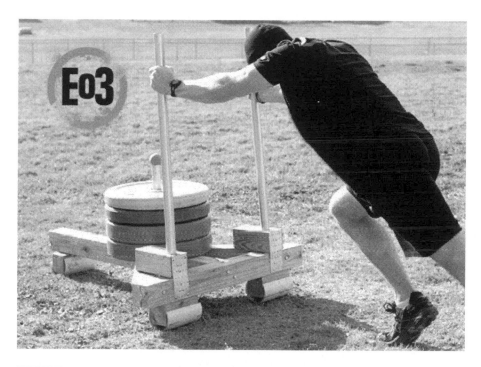

W̲ant to expand your repertoire of handyman skills and get in the best shape of your life all at the same time? Then you, my friend, need to make your very own DIY Prowler. Never heard of a Prowler? Let me tell you what sort of workout you've been missing out on first, and then I'll show how you can make your own with some 4x4s, pipe, and brackets.

What Is a Prowler?

A Prowler is basically a sled that you stack weight on and push around for exercise. But the Prowler isn't just another push or pull workout sled. The different variations and workout combinations you can perform with a Prowler are almost endless, making it an amazing strength and conditioning tool.

Depending on which variations and movements you use, the Prowler is great for conditioning and endurance workouts or for strengthening your core, arms, and lower body. There aren't too many conditioning tools that exist in this world that have the power to work your whole body like the Prowler. A few quick intervals with this thing and you will feel like you ran five miles and completed a load of heavy squats.

The Prowler was made popular by some of the world's top strength training coaches like Dave Tate and Louie Simmons. These coaches learned that any lifting program, if not coupled with appropriate muscle conditioning, prevents athletes from reaching their full potential. Athletes that want to compete at an elite level will need an elite level of conditioning to get through their training.

With CrossFit® exploding in popularity, we have seen a huge shift in the world of fitness. Movements and lifts that were once reserved for Olympians and powerlifters are now being performed by your average CrossFitter. And equipment that was once used only by elite athletes (like the Prowler) is being incorporated into the fitness regimens of more and more average folks.

The problem with some of this cool new fitness equipment is that it can cost you an arm and a leg. For example, buying a heavy-duty Prowler will run you anywhere from $250–$800 at most fitness stores. But with an investment of just fifty bucks, you can build your very own this weekend.

Alright, enough chitchat. Let's start building your Prowler.

Step 1 : Go shopping

Now, before you run out and buy everything on the list, make sure you read through this entire chapter first. I left some things optional. This could make your project easier or cheaper depending on your specific situation. The items on the equipment list with a star have options.

Materials Needed

- (2) - 8' 4×4s
- (1) - 10' metal conduit pipe - 1¼"in diameter★ (or other pipe options that do not involve cutting)
- (10) - 5/16"lag screws 6"(1 extra just in case)
- (1) - Box of flat edge screws 1–1½"
- (1) - 2' PVC section 4" diameter★ (other options available)
- Masonry circular cutoff blade for cutting metal and PVC★ (only if you plan to cut the pipe yourself)

Brackets

- (2) - 6"flat brackets
- (2) - Hurricane bracket straps
- (6) - 90-degree brackets
- (4) - 45-degree brackets (adjustable angle)

Step 2: Cutting the 4x4s

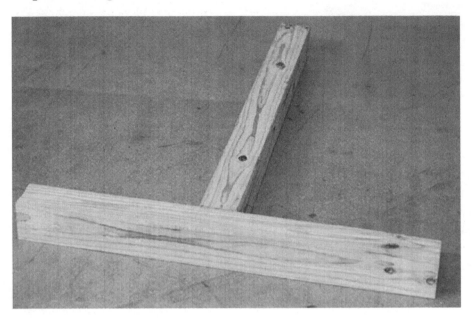

First, we will be cutting the 4x4s for the basic pieces we will use to make the sled. This step includes a majority of the 4x4 cuts; however, there will be more cutting later.

Cut the following:

- (1) - 43-inch piece (used for T-shape)

- (1) - 36-inch piece (used for T-shape)

- (3) - 7-inch pieces (used for the "runners" on the bottom of the sled)

- (2) - 8½-inch pieces (used for support on top of the sled)

Step 3: Boring holes

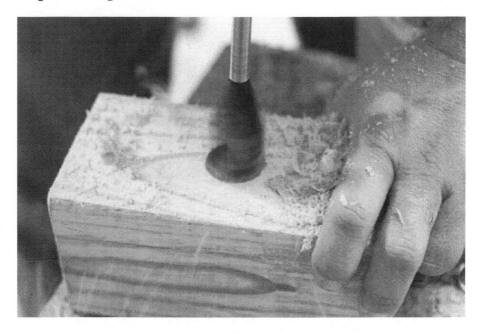

We'll be boring 1½-inch holes in the 4x4 for our pipe. To do this job, you'll need a 1½"hole boring drill bit.

Bore the following holes:

- In the 36-inch piece: 2 holes. Each hole should be 7-inches from each end.

- In the 43-inch piece: 1 "halfway hole." Hole should be 29 inches from one end. DO NOT DRILL ALL THE WAY THROUGH!

- In the two 7-inch pieces: Bore a hole halfway through, directly in the center. DO NOT DRILL ALL THE WAY THROUGH!

- In the two 8½-inch pieces: Bore a hole 2 inches from all the way through.

Step 4: Pipe cutting

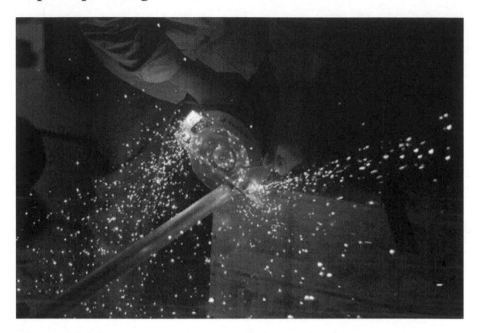

Wow, fire! Don't be scared of some sparks. However, if you do feel uncomfortable cutting pipe you may want to buy the pre-cut galvanized pipe. Yeah, I cut it in the dark for a cool effect. Don't try cutting in the dark at home!

A few notes: The pipe I used is a 1¼-inch conduit pipe that comes in 10-foot sections. It's easy to cut and super cheap. It's plenty strong for this project too. If you don't want to cut pipe, you can buy the smaller sections of galvanized pipe, but it will cost more. You can purchase a skill saw blade for two to three dollars that cuts conduit pipe.

Cut the following:

- (2) - 43-inch pieces
- (1) - 18-inch piece

Step 5: Putting it all together and bracing

Now we take all of your pieces and put them together, and add brackets and some wooden braces.

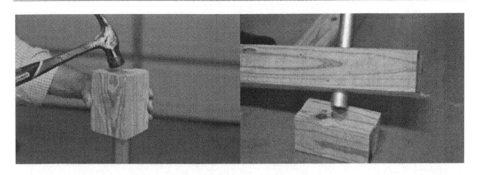

First, we will seat the pipes through all the wood. Take two 43-inch pieces of pipe and thread them through both holes on the 36-inch and two of your 7-inch wood pieces. This may take some tapping on the pipe to get it through. If so, use a piece of 4x4 on top of the pipe and then use a hammer on top of the wood. This will keep the pipe from getting damaged.

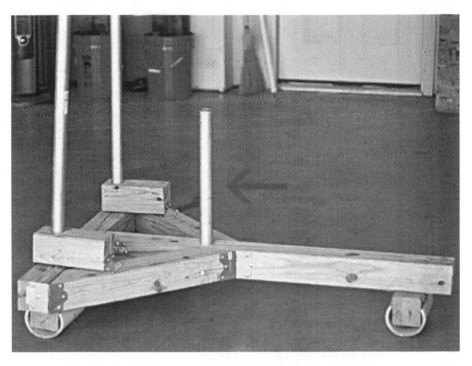

Next, put your 18-inch pipe through the "halfway hole" on your 43-inch piece of 4x4 (See arrow on my completed sled). This is where the weight will be held. Once the project is complete, I recommend putting a tennis ball or racquetball on top of the pipe for safety.

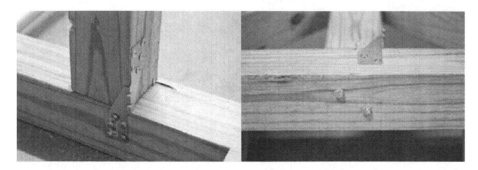

Next, we will secure the T-shape. The top of the T is your 36-inch 4x4. Place the 43-inch 4x4 perpendicular to the 36-inch 4x4 to form the T-shape. Fasten the two beams together with two hurricane brackets and two 6-inch bolts as shown above. One hurricane strap goes on top and the other will go on the opposite side and on the bottom. This will secure and minimize any torque on the T-shape. The bolts will be 45-degree angles from one another. Note: Pre-drill a hole then screw in the bolt.

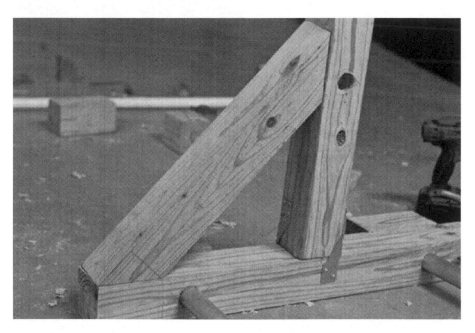

Now we have the basic structure and it is time to add braces. You will need to cut two 24-inch pieces of 4x4 at an angle that will fit your sled.

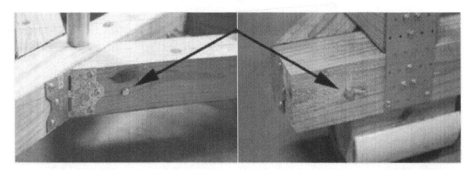

After cutting the two brace beams, secure them with bolts. (Note: In the picture you'll notice I have the brackets screwed on. I took this picture after I completed the project. We haven't gotten to bracket installation yet.)

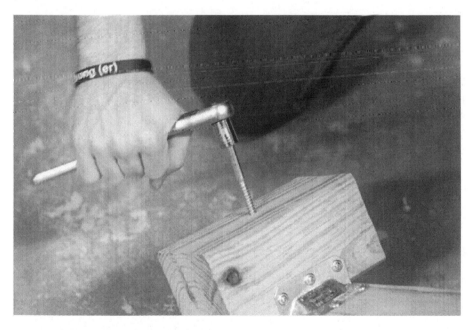

Now secure the third 7-inch runner piece to the bottom 43-inch 4x4 towards the end. Screw in a 90-degree bracket on each side of the 7-inch runner piece. Note: Pre-drill hole.

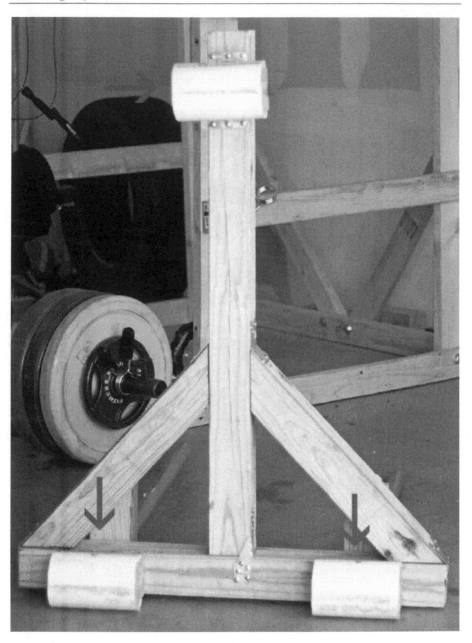

Here's where and how the three 7-inch runner pieces are placed on the bottom of my Prowler. (Ignore the PVC pipe. We'll be adding that in a bit.)

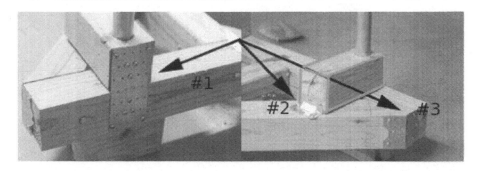

Flip your Prowler so it's resting on the runner pieces. Slide an 8½-inch 4x4 down the pipe (outlined in orange) Add a flat bracket to connect the 8½-inch and 36-inch 4x4s (Arrow #1). Add a 90-degree bracket between the 8½-inch and the angled 24-inch 4x4s (Arrow #2). Add a 45-degree adjustable angle bracket to connect the 36-inch and 24-inch angled 4x4s (Arrow #3). Repeat on the other end.

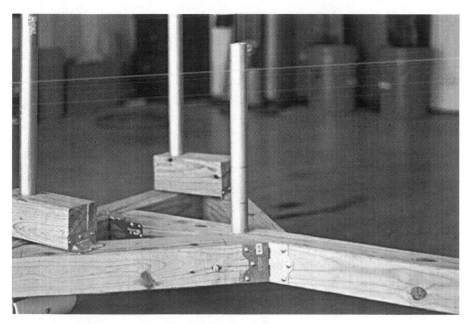

Your sled is basically complete. All we need now is a surface for it to glide on.

Step 6: PVC cutting

I used PVC on my 7-inch runner pieces, and it has worked out great. However, I only use my sled on grass. I like the PVC because it's easily replaceable if it breaks or gets worn. You can really get creative here. You could use a bucket cut in half to secure to the bottom or you could use those hard plastic furniture movers. I am currently using PVC and am enjoying it, but I may try some other material in the future. Just keep that in mind.

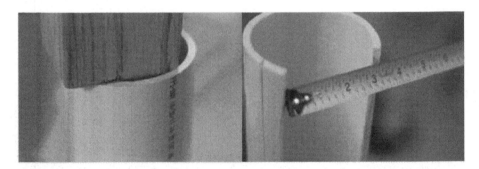

Put the 4x4 at the edge of the PVC to measure the width for your cut. Add tick marks where the wood meets the PVC edge. Draw a perfectly straight line down the edge of the PVC. These will be your cut lines.

After you have the center cut out, you will then cut the PVC into three 7½-inch pieces.

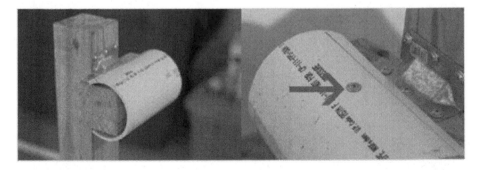

Take your three PVC pieces and slide them on the wood runners. Pre-drill a hole in the PVC and into the wood. Secure the PVC to the wood with flat screws, the longer the better. (See arrow.)

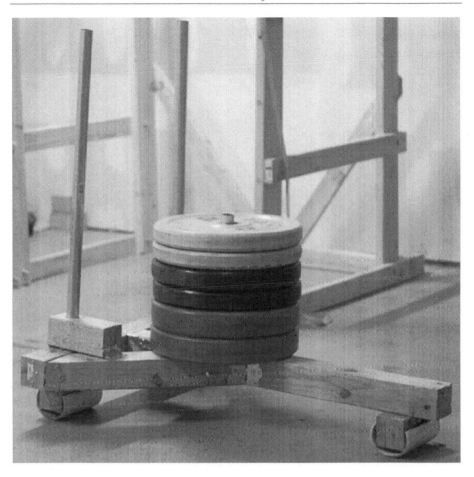

Now you have a fully functional sled!

Now Go Use It!

Chapter 17

DIY Pull-up Bar in 10 Minutes

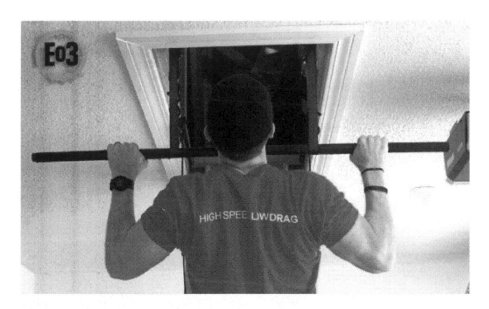

First, a little backstory.

My family and I moved from Texas to Florida and I, of course, had to disassemble the DIY power rack for the move.

When we moved into our new house, I was itching to start using my garage gym right away, but I didn't want to take the time to reassemble the power rack, which, coincidentally, is the only way I can normally do pullups. This was my temporary solution, a very quick DIY pull-up bar.

What You Need to Know

- **Time**: 10 minutes or less

- **Cost**: Free (depends on what you have around the garage)

- **Difficulty**: Insanely easy

A few more things to note:

- This *is not* a great solution for kipping pull-ups.

- This *is* a great solution for muscle-ups and ring dips (as shown below).

- This really only works if A) You have attic access and B) said attic access is in your garage.

Step 1: Gather/buy material

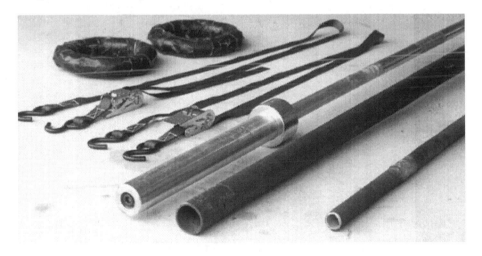

Gather the following

- (2) - Rings (optional)

- (1) - 1″ galvanized pipe (length does not matter)

- (2) - Ratchet tie-down straps

- (1) - Bar of some sort

A little explanation:

- Rings are optional, while this pull-up bar is only a temporary solution for me, this is my permanent solution to muscle-ups and ring dips.

- Bar of some sort. I actually use a black pipe (as seen in picture above) that goes in my attic. You can buy a galvanized pipe from Home Depot or Lowe's, or if you have an extra barbell, you can use that as well. I chose to use the barbell in the DIY pics, simply because most people looking to do this project will have a barbell (I hope).

Step 2: Open attic & place bar

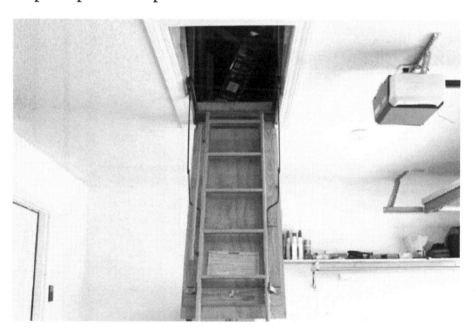

Clear out your crap.

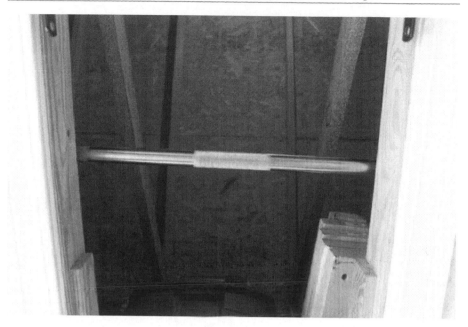

Place bar.

Tips:

- Use a long bar. You want the bar to rest on as many horizontal support beams in your attic as possible. Doing so will ensure that the weight is distributed across multiple support beams, and that you won't end up on the floor of your garage with half your attic on top of you. A barbell is about 7 feet, and the black bar I use is about 8 feet and reaches many support points in my attic.

- Be safe getting the bar in the attic. Get a friend to help you if you can. If not, just make sure you are stable. I got it up there by myself no problem.

Step 3: Hang straps/bar/rings

Measure out the length you will need to be able to do pull-ups without smacking your face into the ceiling. You can also do pull-ups to where your head is going into the attic every rep.

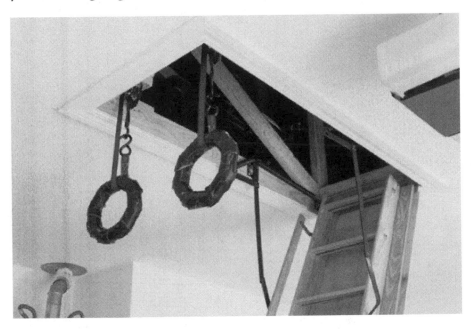

If you will be using this setup for muscle-ups and ring dips, it is more important to get the length of the straps right for the muscle-ups than it is the pull-ups.

Step 4: Use it!

The best way to use it is to half close the attic.

Optional Step 5: Employ infant helper

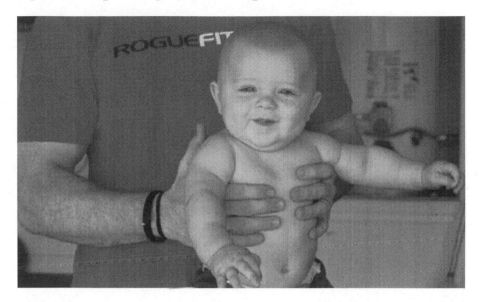

Little man was out in the garage for the entire project (with motherly su-
pervision), which really just goes to show you how quick, easy, and safe
this project is.

Chapter 18

How to Build a Mini Deadlift Jack

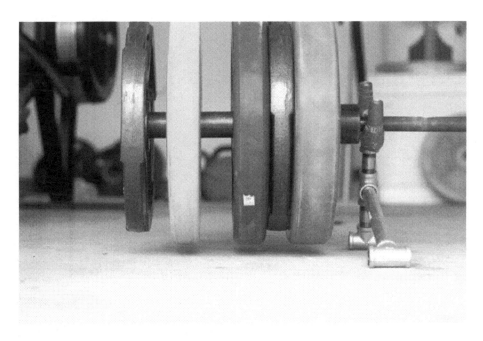

You know what's not fair? The fact that when you bench press, strict press, squat, and do many other lifts, your barbell rests nicely on a rack, making removing weight and adding weight a breeze.

What about the other lifts?

You know, the ones that start from the ground?

Why does it have to be so hard to load and unload the barbell; it's not fair.

Ok, ok, it's either not fair or we are all inherently lazy—even when working out. Either way, let's even the playing field with these from-the-ground lifts!

Please welcome the mini deadlift jack to your DIY arsenal!

This project almost happened on accident. I ended up in the plumbing section of a hardware store, started looking at some pipe and within 10 minutes I had pretty much assembled this project in the store.

It's up to you to decide if making your loading and unloading of a barbell a little bit easier is worth $30, but it's a fun and easy project. I have found this little tool very useful, especially with really heavy deadlifts.

What You Need to Know

- **Time**: 10 minutes

- **Cost**: Around $30

- **Difficulty**: Easy. If you can't do this one, there is no hope for you.

Step 1: Buy mini deadlift jack supplies

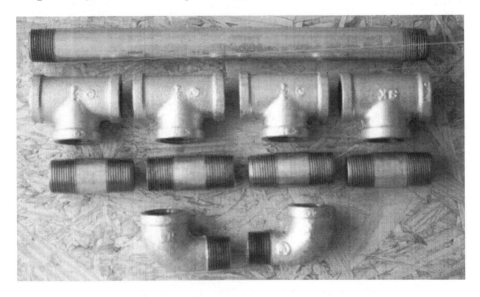

- (1) - ¾"x 12"galvanized pipe

- (4) - ¾"galvanized T-pieces

- (4) - ¾"x 2½"galvanized pipe

- (2) - ¾"elbow joints

Optional: Duct tape (you probably already have this)

Duct tape: This is optional because the mini deadlift jack is 100 percent useable without the application of any sort of tape. However, it doesn't take a rocket scientist to realize that metal rubbing on metal is not usually a good thing (that's why we have oil in our cars). So, over time, without the tape, the mini deadlift jack will rub, scuff, and scratch your barbell.

Step 2: Assemble main mini deadlift jack structure

After writing this, I realize the text can be more confusing than necessary. Just look at the pictures, it is extremely simple. Putting it into words makes it more complex than it seems.

Complete the Following

Connect your 12-inch piece into a T-piece.

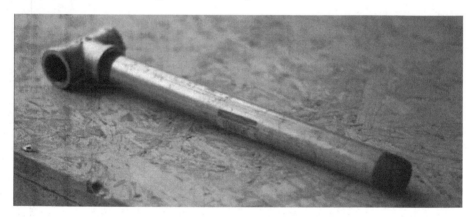

Connect another T-piece on the opposite end of the 12-inch pipe, with the top T-hole facing up and down.

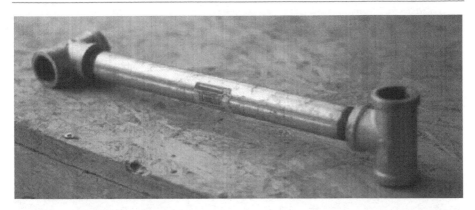

Connect a 2½-inch piece into the previously stated T-piece, pointed downward. Connect your final T-piece onto the end of your 2½-inch piece, and make sure that it is parallel to the T-piece at the end of the mini deadlift jack. If they are not perfectly parallel, and tight, it will make for a wobbly mini deadlift jack.

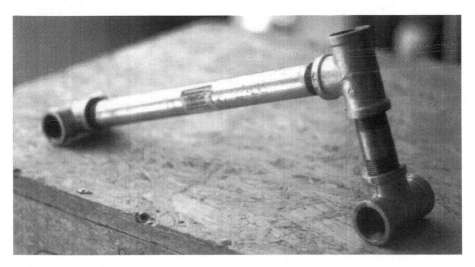

Add a 2½-inch piece to the top of the upward facing T-piece.

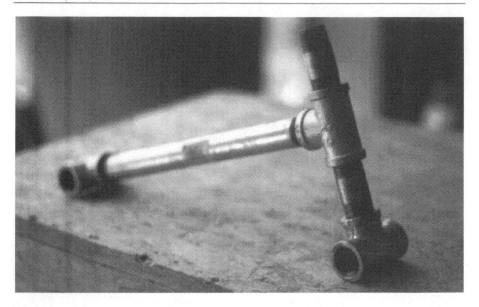

Now we have the main structure for the mini deadlift jack. Make sure all of the pieces are extremely tight. Also, I'll say it again, make sure the two T-pieces that are touching the ground are very tight and perfectly level with each other.

Step 3: Construct the mini deadlift jack weight holder

Very easy step here: Take a T-piece and attach both elbow joints so that they are tight and parallel. Next, connect your last 2½-inch pieces and screw them into the elbow joints.

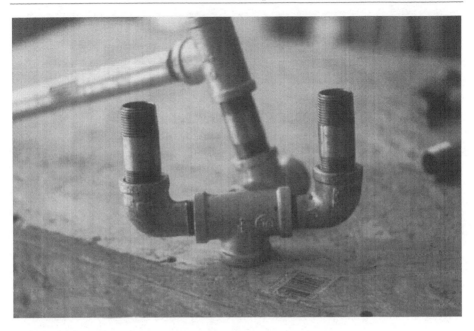

Simply screw this piece into the mini deadlift jack main structure and you are pretty much done. If you want to add the tape, it is easiest to add the tape before you screw it onto the mini deadlift main structure. That will leave you with a finished product as seen below.

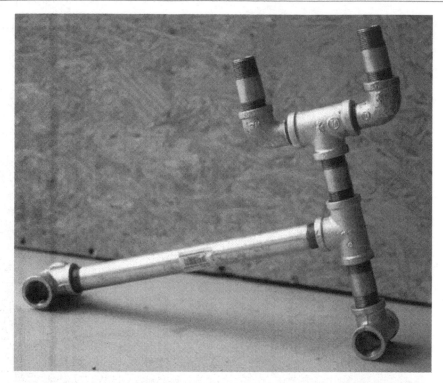

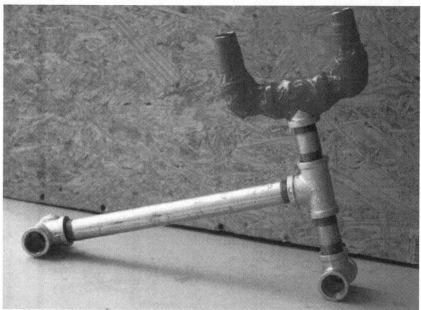

Step 4: Use your mini deadlift jack!

It is very easy to use, but here are some things to know before you try it out.

Place the mini deadlift jack firmly on the bar where the elbow joint and 2½-inch piece connect, and then on the ground.

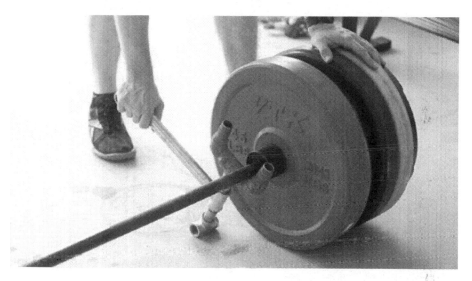

Carefully apply force to the lever and do not get your finger crushed under this thing! I normally guide the barbell with my other hand by putting it on the sleeve of the barbell, just to make sure there is no catastrophic failure. So far so good.

Note: Since there is such a wide gap in the barbell-holding piece of our mini deadlift jack, the bar will slide from the top to the bottom. Don't be alarmed! This is where the duct tape really comes in handy. It slows the bar from sliding and will make sure the bar is safe.

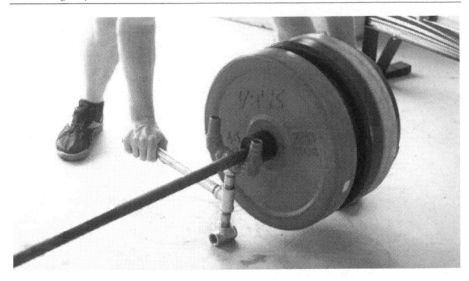

Lastly, even up the score with those racked position lifts! Easily add and remove your weight.

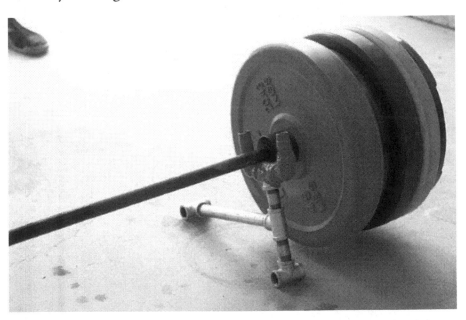

There should be just enough clearance, no matter if you have bumper plates or iron.

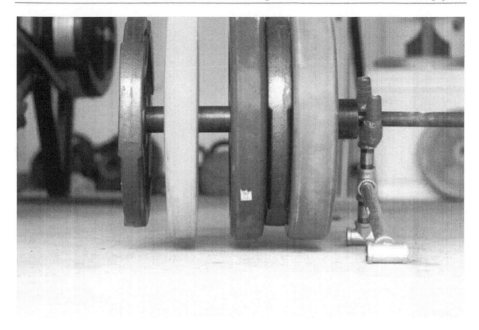

If you just want an alternative. Yes, rolling your weight onto a 2.5-pound plate works well for racking and unracking your weight too. But it's not near as cool.

Chapter 19

How to Build a Kettlebell in 36 Seconds

What You Need to Know

- **Time**: 36 seconds

- **Cost**: $20 or less

- **Difficulty**: Insanely easy

Awhile back, I trained my parents online. They have minimal equipment and aren't really in the market to buy anything serious.

I designed a workout for them that involved kettlebell swings. I knew they did not own a kettlebell so I recommended using an old milk jug filled with sand or even a laundry detergent canister for the swings.

They used the laundry detergent bottle, but they said it wasn't great.

So there had to be a solution—DIY!

First, let me say this is a "simple kettlebell," designed for kettlebell swings only, and on top of that, primarily Russian kettlebell swings.

If you are interested in Pavel Tsatsouline's kettlebell workouts, I suggest building the more elaborate homemade KB's or even purchasing your own. This version is quick, easy, and a very cheap way to throw kettlebell swings into your training immediately. As long as you know what this version should be used for—we can now get started.

Step 1: Buy material

Buy the following

- (1) - 1"galvanized flange
- (1) - 1"galvanized T-shape
- (2) - 5"long x 1"diameter galvanized pipe pieces
- (1) - 6"long x 1"diameter galvanized pipe pieces
- (2) - 1"galvanized end caps

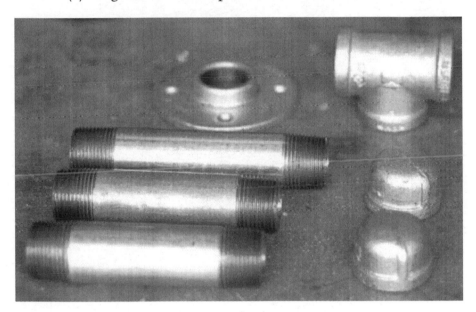

All materials used.

Step 2: Put it all together

Get ready to start your stopwatch! Also, don't blink or you may miss it!

In 36 seconds or less, here we go:

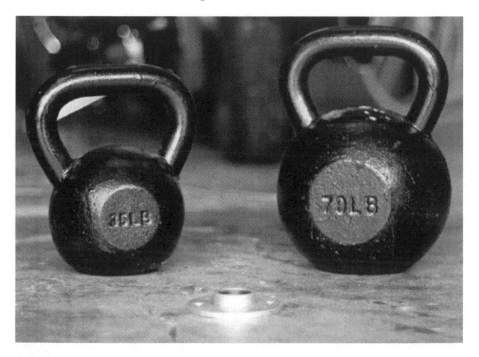

Start with the flange.

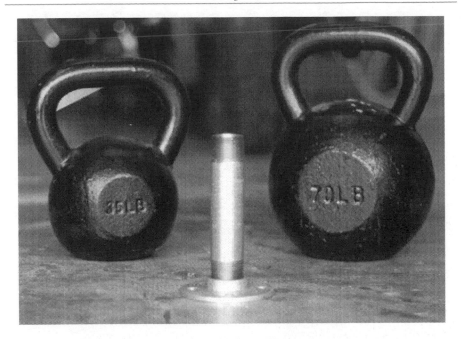

The 6-inch piece screws into the flange.

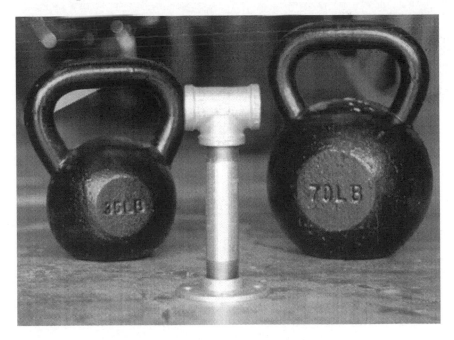

T-shape goes on top of the 6-inch piece.

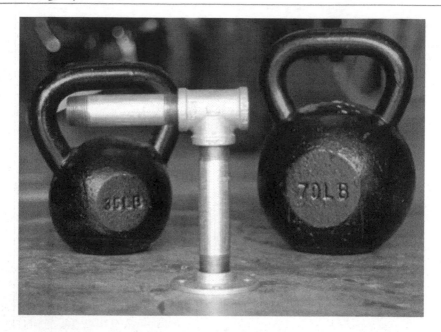

The 5-inch piece goes into T-shape (1).

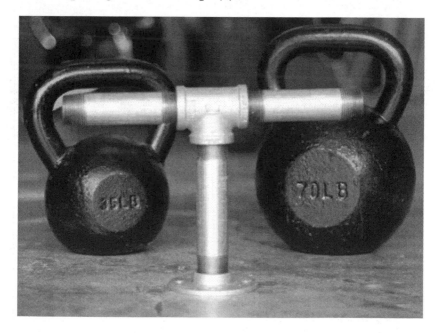

The 5-inch piece goes into T-shape (2).

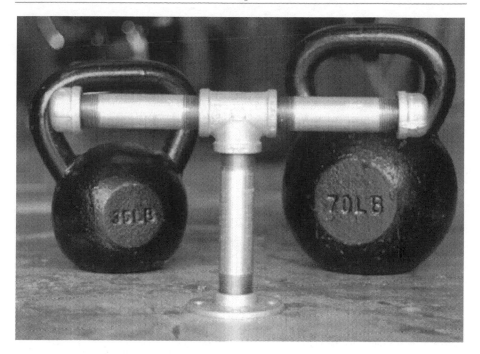

End caps go on 5-inch pieces. Kettlebell complete!

Stop time! How long did it take you?

Step 3: Remove bottom flange and add weight plates of your choice (5 pounds, 10 pounds).

Step 4: Swing.

Step 5: Get in shape knowing you are not part of the fitness "norm."

Notes:

- If you feel this is too wide for your legs, or hands, you can buy smaller pieces for your handles.

- If you need to add more plates but don't want a larger plate size, just buy a longer vertical pipe and stack more.

- Plates won't be a snug fit. Use duct tape to widen diameter and dampen the noise.

Suggested workouts with your new KB

Recruit

3 rounds for time

- 10 reps, kettlebell sumo dead lift high pulls
- 10 reps, kettlebell swings

Established

3 rounds for time

- 400-meter run
- 1.5 pood kettlebell swing x 21
- Pull-ups, 12 reps

Competitor

For time (if you have built our other projects)

50-40-30-20 and 10-rep rounds of

- Wall ball shots, 20-pound ball
- Box jump, 24-inch box
- Kettlebell swings, 1.5 pood

Like I said there are more elaborate versions you could create, but this is quick, easy, and cheap.

Chapter 20

Homemade Squat and Bench Press Stand

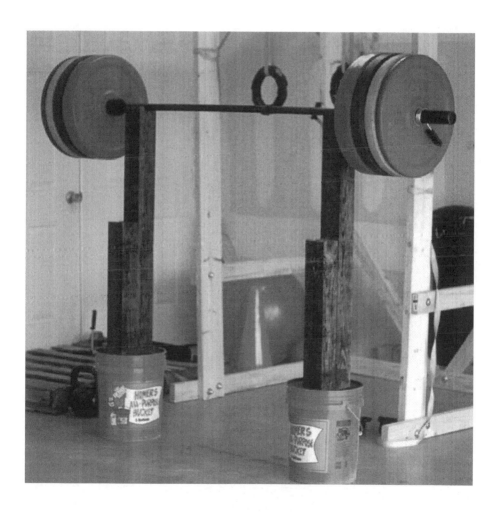

What You Need to Know

- **Cost**: $31

- **Time**: 2 hours

- **Difficulty**: Medium

Equipment for Squatting, Benching, and Pressing

Materials Needed

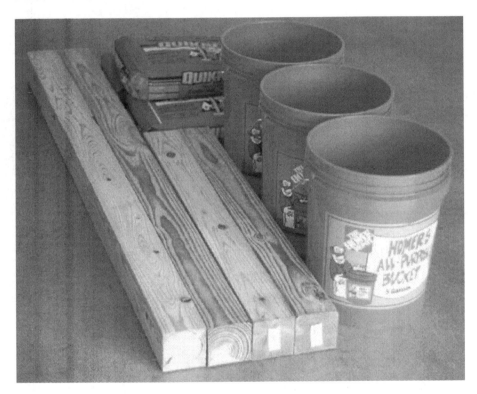

- (3) - 5-gallon buckets

- (3) - 50-pound bags of QUIKRETE (fast setting)

- (2) - 8-foot 4x4s

Step 1: Go to your local hardware store and pick up your items

At Home Depot, they will make two cuts for free. I had them cut the 8-foot piece at 5 feet, which gave me two 5-foot pieces and two 3-foot pieces. Take into account how high you want your stands. I originally had it at 60 inches (or 5 feet), but decided I wanted it a little shorter after I started the project so I had to make two more cuts. I ended up with two 3-foot pieces and two 55-inch pieces. I am five feet eleven.

Step 2: Make your V-cuts

If you have a skill saw, put it at 45 degrees and make the cut. This step was far more complicated than it needed to be, but if you mess it up, you are screwed. If you are unsure how to make a V-cut, please refer to the images in this chapter. If you are using a handsaw, just draw a V and cut accordingly.

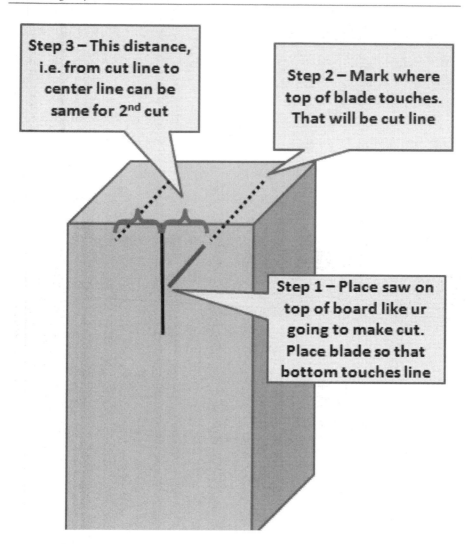

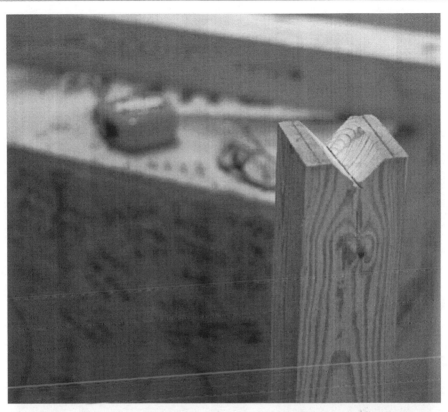

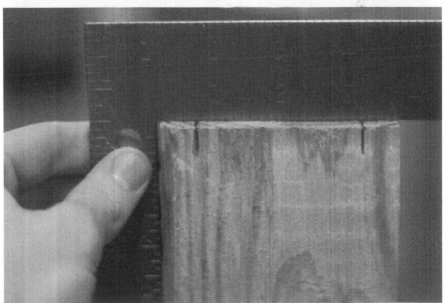

Step 3: Cement work

There are not as many pictures of these steps because it is a little messy and involved.

There are directions on the back of QUIKRETE for setting a fence post. DO NOT use those directions. Mix all of your cement in your third bucket; that is why you bought it.

Cement Tips:

- Mix small amounts of the bag of dry cement with water, until you eventually use the whole bag.

- Do not mix more than one bag at a time.

Put your fence posts together. I duct-taped them together and placed them in the bucket. Once you have it mixed according to the instructions on the back of the bag you can now pour it from the mixing bucket to around your fence post. It helps if someone will hold the post while you pour. You do not want any cement under the post—that is why it goes in first.

Recap:

- Duct-tape smaller and large post together

- Put in one of the dry buckets

- Mix cement

- Pour mixed cement around post

- Let dry

Use a level to make sure it is straight. The cement should be thick enough to hold it upright with no assistance. Just make sure you make it straight before the cement sets.

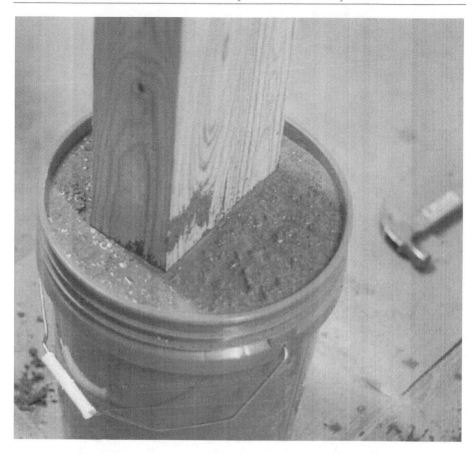

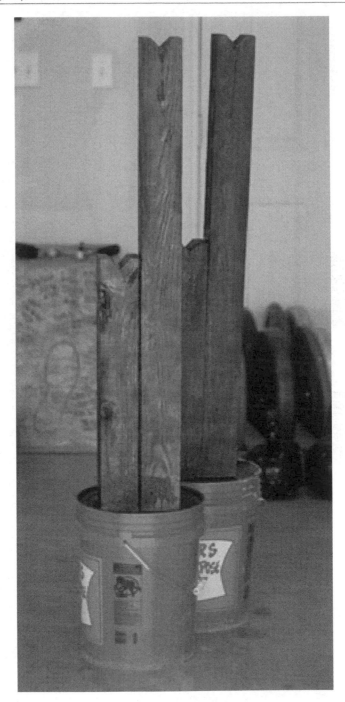

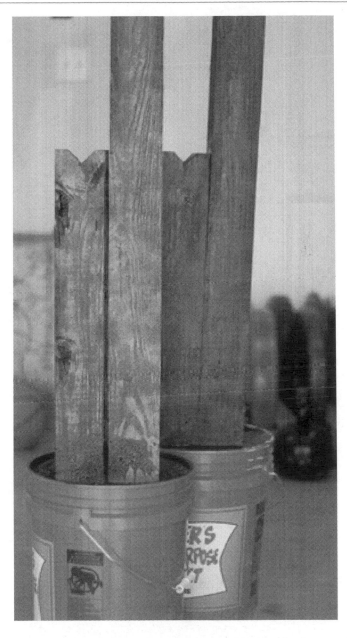

That's it! I had some old spray paint I wanted to get rid of, so I added that in at the end.

Chapter 21

Build Your Own Rings

Materials Needed

- (16) - ½"45-degree elbow joints
- (1) - 5' PVC pipe ½"diameter
- (1) - Roll of gorilla tape
- (1) - Can of PVC cement
- (3) - Canisters of heavy-duty Liquid Nails (optional)

Step 1:

- Cut (16) - 2-inch pieces of PVC off your long PVC pipe.
- Put PVC cement on the inside of a 45-degree elbow joint and on the end of one of your 2-inch pieces.
- Build the rings into halves that look like this:

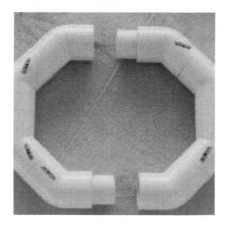

Optional Instructions:

- Fill the inside of each half with heavy-duty Liquid Nails and let dry for 10 minutes.

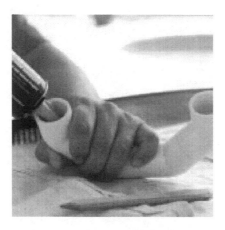

Step 2:

- Put the two halves together with PVC cement; let dry for 20 minutes.

- Wrap Gorilla Tape around all the connections, and then around the rest of the ring.

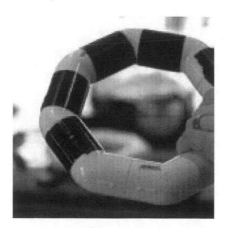

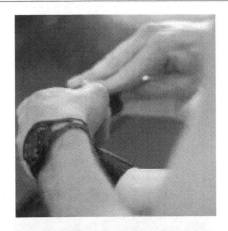

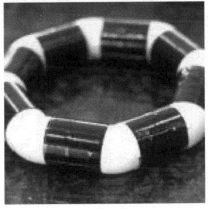

Now you have your own rings!

I connect mine to tie-down straps used for trucks (the big ones that can be cranked down for different lengths).

They work great! Now go get some muscle-ups!

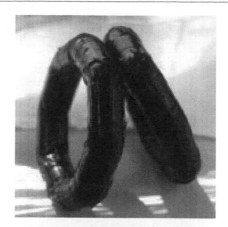

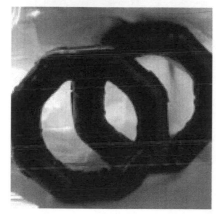

Section Three

Train like a Pro

Chapter 22

A Primer on Programming and Being an Athlete

In the first section of this book we opened your mind to garage gyms, being a Garage Gym Athlete, and starting your journey down this path.

In the second section, I gave you a dozen DIY projects you could use that could quite literally change your life, and if you didn't DIY, you at least got a good idea of what to buy.

Now, in the third section we talk about training, or more specifically we talk about programming, which is simply how you put your program design together to meet your goals. But first I have to say one thing: I hate crappy programs. My goal for the past decade has been to figure out how to create the perfect program. But here's what I've found—it doesn't exist!

I spend hours writing, calculating, and planning my own programming each month. I need it to work, to keep me interested, and it has to be fun! While I have found the perfect program doesn't exist, I have also gained a new skill that serves me extraordinarily well, and serves those who I coach. That is, I know how to program my own training very well.

In this section of the book, I want to at least give you an idea of how to be your own programmer, and leave you with some training and ideas to get you started.

In the last couple of years I have coached hundreds of athletes to meet their goals, and I am finding what I have been working on works for a lot of different types of people:

- CrossFit® competitors

- Stay-at-home moms

- Endurance athletes

- Special operators

- Obstacle racers

- And Garage Gym Athletes!

In the next chapter I will show you the programming framework I created, which makes programming work for anyone! Soon, you'll be on your way to acquiring similar programming skills. It takes time, effort, and planning but acquiring the programming skill will serve you well for the rest of your life.

Remember, I want you to succeed in the long run and not have some three-week spurt of motivation.

Because do you want to know the truth? You may never reach that goal. Why? Well, the real *why* comes down to something as simple as time. You don't have enough time, you don't use that time properly, and you know how life goes. It's hard to set a huge goal and see it to the end.

People jump from program to program, or never see a program to the end and only ever see a fraction of the results they truly want.

But it is possible—to reach your goal. I'm living proof that *you* can get an absurd amount of amazing training done in less than 60 minutes. Honestly, I don't have a lot of time. I put time with my wife and kids ahead of fitness every day. Sometimes that means a workout doesn't happen.

It's been years since I started my garage gym. It's become a lifestyle for me. It's pretty funny to see the look on people's faces when I tell them I run a fitness business, but I haven't been to a gym in years. But it hasn't always been a lifestyle. And honestly, it was hard to figure things out at first. Right off the bat, I was a lot of things:

- I was my own coach.

- I was my own accountability partner.

- I was my own nutritionist.

- I was my own programmer.

- I was the engineer behind all my DIY equipment.

- I was the janitor.

- I was EVERYTHING!

At the beginning, I was also transitioning from the bodybuilder mindset (bench on Monday, legs on Tuesday, etc.) to becoming a strength and conditioning athlete. The transition was like drinking water from a fire hose. There was so much to learn! Now, fast-forward to today: I feel there is always more to learn, but I finally feel like I know what I am doing.

What am I doing? I'm an athlete! I'm not a professional, I'm not on a team, but I am an athlete. How do you become an athlete?

The quickest way to succeed in health and fitness is to act like an athlete. Act like this stuff is an actual priority, let your friends and family know it IS a priority, and get serious.

- Follow programming for more than three weeks.

- Take your nutrition seriously.

- Get serious!

Working out in your garage makes you more serious than most, so act like it.

Becoming an athlete has done a lot for me:

- I've been able to run a marathon, ride in a 100-mile bike race, and I completed a Spartan Beast.

- I've gone well below sub-6 on a mile, and deadlifted three times my body weight.

But most of all, acting like an athlete has given me the motivation to keep at it day after day!

And we have now assembled a community, around this singular idea. Garage Gym Athlete is our fully comprehensive training system and community to make powerful and athletic human beings. If you know you want to be an athlete, but feel lost when it comes to programming, this is the perfect fit.

It is like joining a pro team. There is a head coach. An order to the program. Interaction. Demos. Literally everything you need. This isn't just a bunch of random workouts thrown together. It's a system that will take your training to the next level.

No, you don't have to join our community, and honestly, I am going to try and teach you some of my secrets in this section of the book. But it may just be a perfect fit for you.

Now, let's get started on how to train like the pros.

Chapter 23

Save Your Time: Block Programming

Let me show you the programming technique I've been using to fully optimize my time and the time of numerous athletes who are on a "time budget."

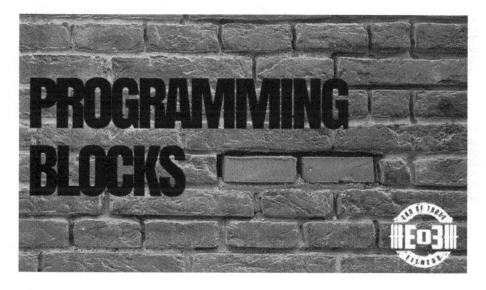

The challenge in any workout program is doing everything *you* want to do in the time that *you* have.

I know one of the biggest struggles for most people is finding the time to train and work out.

Or if you have the time, not being able to execute everything you want in that time frame, which is typically an hour, or less.

So what are your options?

You could work faster to get it all done, you could have someone help you program more efficient training, or you can do what I do.

Program your training in blocks.

Programming and planning your workouts in blocks will lead to more efficient training, help you get more done, and you won't ever stress out from having a workout last too long or, worse, having to cut a workout short.

Whether it is CrossFit® programming, strength programming, Cross-Fit® and strength programming, endurance programming . . . it doesn't matter.

Programming in blocks steals the idea from the Zone diet where one "block" is equivalent to a certain measure of protein, carbohydrates, or fat.

In our discussion on programming, our blocks are our time.

Specifically, one block is equal to 10 minutes. But let's start with why.

Why program in blocks?

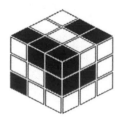

Ideal training is kind of like eating all your fruits and vegetables every day.

You really want to, you know the benefits, and sometimes you even get it done.

But a lot of the times it just doesn't happen. Right?

Let's look at ideal CrossFit® programming: Because ideally, aside from the main parts of your training like strength and conditioning, you should also be developing skills, working on weaknesses, doing mobility work, having a thorough warm-up and cool down, etc.

But is there enough time for all that?

Not really.

Unless you program in blocks.

Programming your daily workouts in 10-minute blocks will help you get as close to ideal training as possible, and without leaving any elements out.

How to Program in Blocks

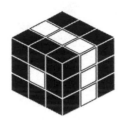

A programming block is equal to 10 minutes.

So, say you have an hour to work out; that means you have 5 blocks.

No, I didn't just have a mathematical stroke.

- You have five 10-minute blocks, which equals 50 minutes.
- And you have one 10-minute block (for every hour of training) called the "invisible block."

The invisible block is not yours for training. It factors in transition time, racking weight, getting out equipment, brief rests, etc.

You have to factor in one invisible block for every hour of training. Trust me. If you make a 6-block training schedule for an hour, it will take you 1 hour and 10 minutes. Try me.

Likewise, if you want to train for two hours, you have 10 training blocks and two invisible blocks.

Now you've got the concept. Next.

What does a block look like?

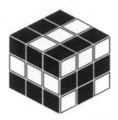

A block is anything you can fit into 10 minutes, which is one of most things.

If it would take 20 minutes, that's obviously two blocks.

Example blocks

- You could make your warm-up and cool down each half blocks (for a total of one block)

- Working sets of strength would be about one block

- Volume work in strength would be one block

- A metcon would be one block, and occasionally two blocks (20 min AMRAP)

- A mobility session is one block

- One mile run is about one block

- Murph is 3–5 blocks

- EMOM lifting should be about one block

- A long run is 3–5 blocks

Is this making sense?

It will make sense when I show you an example day.

So let's do that . . .

Example Blocked Training Session

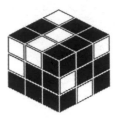

Remember the rules!

- 1 block = 10 minutes
- 1 hour = 5 training blocks + 1 invisible block

That means I have 5 blocks of time to get some stuff done.

What could I do?

Here is a 5-block (or 1-hour) training session in which we get a *ton* of work done, and won't go a second over 60 minutes:

Blocked Training Session:

[Half Block 1]

- General dynamic warm-up

Snatch [Block 2]

- 12 sets of 2 reps @ 60% 1-rep max, performing reps every 45 seconds on the second

Clean & Jerk [Block 3]

- 12 sets of 2 reps @ 60% 1-rep max, performing reps every 45 seconds on the second

Accessory [Block 4]

3 rounds (one round every 3 minutes)

- — Air squat, 25 reps

- — Snatch pull, 5 reps (heavy weight)

- — Toes to bar, 10 reps

General Fitness [Block 5]

- — Zercher walks (heavy) – 10 sets of a 10-meter walk

[Half Block 1]

- — 300 seconds in the front-leaning rest position

And that's it!

Programming in blocks can be a real game changer. If you first start with everything you want to accomplish in a week and then break it out into your blocks, you have a very easy way to plan your training week.

The best part is you will get it all done, you won't run over on time or have to cut workouts short, and you will accomplish some really efficient training!

Chapter 24

A Pro Knows How to Train Alone

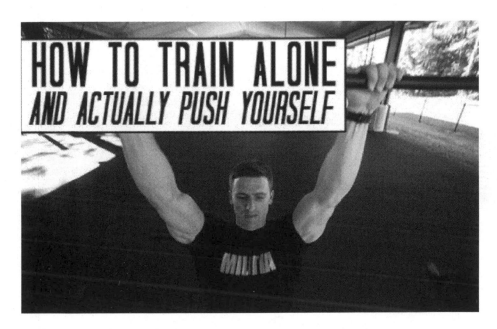

A Garage Gym Athlete will often train alone, and to train alone is to develop a skill, or an art, and it is not simple.

Anybody can walk around the block or go through the motions of a workout alone.

I'm sure you've heard the popular quote, "Eighty percent of success is showing up."

But just *showing up* is not enough.

It builds a habit, but doesn't yield the greatest return.

Do you know how to push yourself when training alone?

I can tell you this.

It's not as easy as saying, "Push yourself!"—and magical workout leprechauns and unicorns get you through it.

No.

But you can put pushing yourself on autopilot with a few simple techniques.

In this chapter, I am going to give you seven techniques you can use to push yourself. Put them in place and you will see the results you want when you train alone.

Like I said, showing up is not enough and you won't get any gold stars from me for *just* completing a workout.

You read that right.

Maybe you feel good breaking a light sweat and burning a few calories, but I call that being a human being. If you want to be better you need to learn to push yourself without a cheerleader, without your favorite music, and without a reward.

Alright, do I have your attention?

I estimate that I have worked out in my garage *alone* well over 1,000 times in the last five years.

And I won't negate having a training partner; they help *tons* and I recommend having a partner if you can, but when you can't, here's what you do . . .

1. Set Meter Goals (once per week)

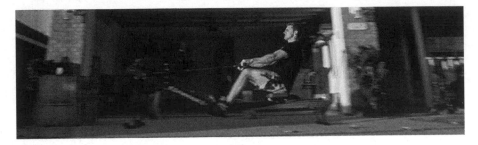

I love interval training.

I think it is one of the best and most effective ways to improve your conditioning.

There is just one problem.

I've tested this as a coach. If I give an athlete many intervals of 30 seconds of work followed by 30 seconds of rest (with no further instruction), the final interval is *wayyyyy* off from the first.

People tend to go out too hard and lose focus over time.

Unless they have a goal, but what should it be?

Here's what you do when planning a 30/30 interval which will have many rounds:

Take your *goal* mile time—say it is 6 minutes flat.

- 6 min = 360 seconds

- Mile = 1600 meters

- m/s = 4.44

- 4.44 x 30 sec would set your minimum distance @ 133 meters per 30 seconds of work.

If it's too easy you aren't doing enough intervals. You can also base it off your 400-meter or 800-meter sprint speeds—it all depends on what you are trying to improve. You can do this all the way up to 5K-race pace with longer work/rest intervals.

It works with rowing, Airdyne, biking, etc.

Do this once a week and stick to your meter goal.

If you don't meet your goal you will apply penalties, which we will talk about in a minute.

Next, we talk about the true motivator—MONEY!

2. Put Your Money Where Your Fitness Is (once per quarter)

This one is my second favorite.

I've never done it but I have a friend who does.

Write a check for $500 (or whatever amount you want, but make it hurt a little) and give it to a trustworthy person who won't listen to your crying and whining.

The Rules are Simple

- *Set a goal:* How many miles you will run, pounds you will lose, a weight you need to squat within 3 months, or a time you'd like to run, etc.

- *Option #1:* Write the check to your friend/spouse and tell them to keep the money if in 3 months you don't achieve your goal.

- *Option #2 (the better option):* Write a check to a charity you *hate*, put it in an addressed envelope with a stamp ready to send, and tell your friend to send the money if you don't meet your goal.

Remember this is about pushing yourself. Pick a challenging goal—like taking 15 seconds off your mile time, or adding 10 pounds to your squat.

Make it hurt.

And if you fail, don't cheat! The money is gone!

3. Benchmark Yourself *Frequently* (once per month)

Now, you need to embrace your competitive nature.

We all have a competitive side, and you will be competing against your greatest enemy—YOURSELF!

If you work out alone, often you need to push yourself more than anyone else because it is too easy to get complacent. If a professional is programming for you, then I'm okay with testing benchmarks every couple of months.

If not, you need to be benchmarking yourself in different areas on a monthly basis.

What benchmarks, you ask? Use the End of Three Fitness benchmarks in the picture below. That is a good place to start.

ELEMENT	COMPETITOR	ESTABLISHED	RECRUIT
Work Time	4+ hours	3+ hours	2+ hours
Deadlift	≥ 2x Bodyweight	≥ 1.5x Bodyweight	≥ 1x Bodyweight
Back Squat	≥ 1.75x Bodyweight	≥ 1.5x Bodyweight	≥ 1x Bodyweight
Front Squat	≥ 1.5x Bodyweight	≥ 1.25x Bodyweight	≥ .75x Bodyweight
Press	≥ 1x Bodyweight	≥ .75x Bodyweight	≥ .5x Bodyweight
Clean	> 1x Bodyweight	≥ .8-.9x Bodyweight	Skill Practice*
Snatch	> 1x Bodyweight	≥ .8-.9x Bodyweight	Skill Practice*
Jerk	> 1x Bodyweight	≥ .8-.9x Bodyweight	Skill Practice*
Eo3 5K	< 40:00	< 50:00	< 60:00
Strict Pull-ups	20+	10-15+	< 10
Strict Dips	20+	10-15+	< 10
2,000m Row	≤ 7:00	≤ 8:00	≤ 9:00
1.5 Mile Run	≤ 9:10	≤ 11:04	≤ 13:01
500m Row	≤ 1:35	≤ 1:50	≤ 2:00
400m Sprint	60 sec. (+/- 5)	75 sec. (+/- 5)	90 sec. (+/- 5)

You should know your maxes and lift off accurate percentages.

If you're scared to max out, get over it.

4. Stick to a Freakin' Program (at least 12 weeks)

If you're not seeing results, I can almost guarantee it is because you aren't sticking to a program.

And if you are, you aren't sticking to it long enough.

I stuck to the End of Three Fitness <u>One Man One Barbell</u> program for 8 MONTHS! Without the slightest deviation, I stuck to the program and added 170 total pounds, across three lifts, to my maxes.

Sticking to one program for 12 weeks, 6 months, or a year is going to push you more *mentally* than it will *anything else*. It can be challenging but in the end it is worth it.

5. Start a Mental Toughness Habit (daily)

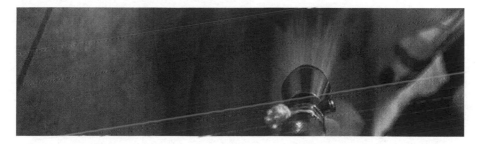

We should have started here.

Because in all honesty, everything I am talking about takes *willpower*.

If you want to build the greatest human strength, you can! Willpower needs training just like anything else, but it needs to be habitual.

I try to do one thing that pushes me mentally each day; something I don't want to do. For me, it's normally a cold shower. Some mornings after working out, I just don't want to take a cold shower (seasonally dependent).

I'll even start with hot and think, *I just don't want to make this water cold.* Anytime I feel like I don't want to, it's almost as if I've trained my hand to adjust the knob before I can finish the thought. Doing this day after day has increased my ability to do things I just don't want to do. It's made me better.

When you wake up in the morning, you are given another opportunity to push yourself, to be better.

Don't squander your time being mediocre or average.

6. Epic Penalty Programming (once per week)

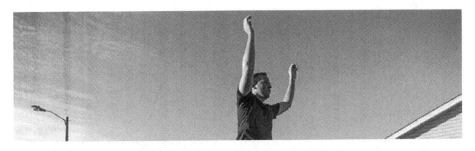

Penalty programming is simple, and you've heard of it. But it takes a lot of self-discipline, which you should be building with your mental toughness habit above.

Example:

- Taking meter goals from above, you could set a 1-burpee-per-meter under your goal penalty, and do them at the end of the workout.

- So if your goal was 133 meters each interval, and in two intervals you did 126 meters and 130 meters, you would do 10 burpees.

Get it? Now, let's make it epic.

It works for a bit, but as you get better at intervals you need to make things a little more epic.

Epic Penalty Programming is this . . .

I was getting good at intervals and would never miss my goals. So I kept increasing my meter goal till I could just *barely* make it—and then I increased it a little bit more.

Then, I set my *epic* penalty at a 1-MILE RUN per meter missed.

There is nothing like tacking on a 3- to 5-mile run at the end of a taxing interval workout to make sure you are pushing yourself.

I only do this to myself once per week.

The trick: COMPLETE the penalties no matter what! Build your willpower.

7. The Iron Mile (once per month)

This is my favorite.

Aside from cold water, I don't know of a better way to push yourself mentally than the Iron Mile.

The point is to walk away from your starting point half mile, and then walk back. That way there is no quitting. Once you make it out there you have to come back, pushing yourself is built into this workout.

Here's the workout:

THE EO3 IRON MILE

FOR TIME...

Walk 1 Mile

The catch—put something on your back, whether it is an empty barbell, a barbell loaded to 185, or empty (or loaded) yoke, but make sure it is metal. No sandbags, medicine balls, or anything comfortable.

A barbell or a yoke. That's it.

Why?

You'll know why about 400 meters in. *You'll want to quit.* You'll start looking for excuses to quit. You'll start blaming me and the stupidity of this programming. You'll feel the pain in your shoulders and upper back, and hey, you may not even get that tired, but you will be pushed.

Once you get past the self-pity and blaming everyone but yourself for lack of mental toughness, you'll know why.

It will be worth it.

Weight *is up to you!* Challenge yourself.

Have fun!

Chapter 25

A Pro Knows How to Wake Up Early

Being a Garage Gym Athlete and turning pro will require discipline in your training; which can mean waking up early.

How to Pass Your First Test of the Day

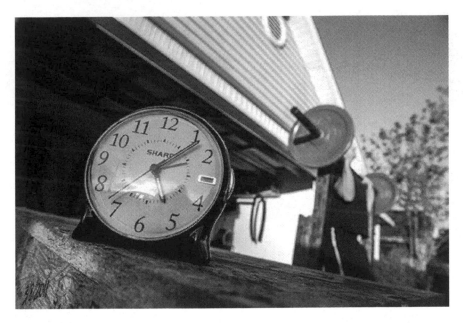

It is said that Chinese rice farmers used to tell one another: "No one who can rise before dawn 360 days a year fails to make his family rich."

I've always loved this quote.

In life, we push ourselves to be better. We want to be better.

We often think of big things when discussing this matter.

Top of mind for most: the goal of a marathon, the mud run and obstacle race, or the goal of lifting more weight than you ever have before.

Goals are great, but if you are going for the "complete overhaul" to achieve your goal, you can forget it.

However, there is a mark, a measure—well, let's call it a test that will determine your success, or failure.

It's a test you most likely took today, and a test you take every day.

There is no grade scale, no nearly passing, no excelling, or extra credit.

The test is pass or fail.

Here it is—what do you do when your alarm clock goes off in the morning?

- Do you spring up, put your feet on the floor and tackle the day?

- Or do you choose comfort over achievement?

It's that simple. Here's why . . .

Discipline equals freedom. — *Jocko Willink*

Sounds contradictory, doesn't it?

But it is true. Discipline does equal freedom.

- If you are disciplined with your money, you have more freedom and options with your money.

- If you are disciplined in health and fitness, you have more freedom in life.

- If you are disciplined with your time, you will have the freedom to do more things with your time.

But do you need to start introducing discipline in every aspect of your life?

Not really.

You need to introduce discipline in one major area that will help every other area of your life.

Do you know what a keystone habit is?

A keystone habit can be the hardest habit to form, but will aid in effortlessly developing numerous good habits.

If you are successful in implementing just *one* keystone habit, you will become a dangerous human being.

It's the lead domino.

The one thing you can do to make everything else easier.

Quick example: If I wake up early, I will work out. When I work out I am happier, I am more productive than I am on the days I don't train. Also, my diet is better because I want to gain from a training session. I will be sure to drink more water, etc.

It's a chain reaction.

I could skirt around the issue and say, "Waking up early is not for everyone."

But aside from medical issues or crazy shift work, there's no real reason you can't wake up early.

For most of us, it is the keystone habit we need.

Don't look for forty-seven ways to change your life. Find the one thing that will have the biggest impact.

Wake up early.

That is the keystone habit that can change your life.

How to Pass the Test (Wake Up Early)

Want to know how to pass your first test of the day?

It's very simple.

Have a reason. Just do it.

There are a few strategies I am about to cover to help those who have an incredibly hard time getting out of bed.

But the real answer is

- Have a Reason

- Just Do It!

Getting up early for the sake of getting up early is kind of weird. But getting up early for a reason is motivational.

With that in mind, if you do struggle with leaving the comforts of bed, I've got you covered.

Here are your tips:

- Ease into it: Set your goal time and work backwards in 30-minute increments. If you wake up at 7 a.m. now and you'd like to start waking up at 5 a.m.—that'll be rough. Chopping two hours off a sleep cycle will make you hate your life. Instead, wake up at 6:30 for a day or two, then 6:00, etc. until you get to your goal time. I am a huge fan of the Band-Aid approach (rip it right off) to most things— so if you want to make a drastic change and have the mental fortitude to do so—do it!

- Go to bed earlier (duh): It should go without saying, but just in case, don't think I am saying wake up earlier and sleep less. I don't thinking sleeping less builds mental toughness. Sleeping less builds poor health not toughness, and makes you a suboptimal human being. Instead, you should go to bed earlier in order to wake up earlier. Let's face it, you probably waste the last hour or two of your day doing frivolous activities.

- Don't think: Your biggest enemy when waking up earlier will be the rational side of your brain. When you are in bed, warm, and still a little tired, any excuse your brain comes up with will be a good one. Don't let that happen. Don't stay in bed long enough to think. Thinking will cripple you (in this case). Get up and go.

- — Alarm at a distance: This is perhaps the easiest tactic you can use on yourself. Put your alarm as far away from you in your room as you can get. A distance that has to be walked to, not reached to, and set the alarm loud. Now, in order to turn that sucker off you have to get up and walk to it. If you are already up and have walked to the other side of the room, you're up! If you get back in bed at this point there is little hope for you.

- — No snooze: Ah, the snooze button. One of the worst inventions/ideas mankind has introduced. What purpose does the snooze button really serve? If you set a time to get up, that should be the time you get up. Why would you build in an hour of snoozing? Interrupted sleep is bad sleep. If you feel like you *need* a snooze, then putting your alarm on the other side of the room is a better option. But don't snooze! Get up!

Alright, that's it!

But remember the real way to start waking up early:

- — Have a Reason

- — Just Do It!

I'll leave you with this . . .

Are you passing your first test of the day?

Then you may just be ready to truly become a Garage Gym Athlete.

Chapter 26

Are You Ready for Fitness Freedom?

Are you ready?

Ready to embrace the underwear freedom?

I've done everything I can do.

You are now ready to work out in your underwear!

Well, I'll leave that optional, and if you decide to, you may want to keep the garage door closed.

As someone with a family who has worked out solely in my garage for years, here are my best parting shots for keeping your fitness freedom.

- Make it a lifestyle: Get the family involved and make sure everyone is on the same page. Fitness should not be viewed as an "if I have time" activity. It is a must. The more you treat it like a non-priority, the less it becomes a part of your life. I've always been confused by people who treat health like it's optional. Just because you are not forced to do something, doesn't mean you shouldn't do it.

- Set a *hard* schedule: If you leave your schedule too open and do not have a set time you work out every day, it will not happen. It is that simple. Set your workout time and use your workout time.

- Train with a purpose: This goes back to goals. Why are you training? It is going to be something a little deeper than "lose 10 pounds"? Because that simply will not last. It is not intrinsic enough. Are you training for your family? For your health? Find your reason!

A few more tips

- Find a program and stick to a program.

There are a lot of effective programs out there, but their effectiveness has a 100 percent correlation with your ability to stick with it. If you don't know what you are doing, don't act like it! You will be wasting your time. Pick a program and stick to it.

Must haves

- Video Camera: This is a must, especially if you are just starting out. A good smart phone will work, especially if you get an app like Coach's Eye. You could watch an instructional video 100 times and do what seems and feels right, but after you watch yourself on video you realize you are doing a lot of it incorrectly. Take time and learn the movements correctly.

- Workout Log: You have to keep track of your progress. I always recommend Evernote. It helps because you can use the search function and find out how you did on workout XYZ two years ago.

- Training Library: If you get into Evernote, it would be a good idea to have a huge bank of programs, exercises, and resources to have accessible at all times or simply have a file dedicated to this on your computer's hard drive.

- Goals: If you and a trainer stepped into a gym and you asked your trainer, "What are we doing today?" and he said, "Ehhh, let's play it by ear," what would you say? Set short and long term goals and hold yourself accountable.

- Ability to tell yourself you suck: If you cannot tell yourself you suck, getting better is going to be difficult. If you take a video and you say, "Well it's not too bad," and you think you're finished, you're wrong. You need to critique every little thing you do—right and wrong. Don't beat yourself up, and don't constantly be negative, but hold yourself to a high standard and be honest.

And that's just getting started!

BOTTOM LINE: Take the time and effort to learn how to coach yourself, or you will be wasting your time!

You are now free!

Bonus Chapter 1

Bodyweight Routines

Thirty-one of my favorite *all*-bodyweight workouts:

1. Walking lunge 400 meters

2. 150 burpees, for time

3. 4 rounds

- Run 400 meters

- 50 squats

4. 100-75-50-25 reps

- Sit-ups

- Flutter kicks (4 count)

5. Crouching tiger

- 50 squats

- 25 push-ups

- 50 pistols

- 25 fingertip push-ups

- 50 side lunges

- 25 knuckle push-ups

- 50 walking lunges

- 25 diamond push-ups

6. For time

- 50 flutter kicks
- 50 sit-ups
- Run 400 meters
- 100 flutter kicks
- 100 sit-ups Run
- 400 meters

7. 4 rounds of

- 50 push-ups
- 50 sit-ups

8. As many rounds as possible in 12 minutes of

- 10 push-ups
- 15 sit-ups
- 20-meter walking lunge

9. 21-15-9 reps of

- lunges (each leg, half rep)
- sit-ups
- burpees

10. 5 rounds of

- 50 mountain climbers (4 count)
- 25 sit-ups

11. 5 rounds of

- 100 jumping jacks
- 100 mountain climbers

12. The prison workout

- 20-19-18 . . . 3-2-1

- Burpee

- Walk 25 meters

13. 50 rounds of

- 1 squat

- 1 push-up

- 1 sit-up

- 1 superman

- 1 tuck jump

14. 5 rounds of

- 30 second isometric squat hold

- 20 squats

- 30 seconds isometric leaning rest

- 20 push-ups

15. For time

- 50 jumping jacks

- 50 push-ups

- 50 tuck jumps

- 50 sit-ups

- 50 mountain climbers (50 each leg)

- 50 squats

- 50 jumping jacks

16. 10 rounds

- 30 seconds handstand
- 30 seconds isometric squat
- Score is cumulative time

17. Playing with push-ups

- Run 100 meters
- 20 push-ups
- 5 burpees
- 15 clap push-ups
- 5 burpees
- 10 chest slap push-ups
- 5 burpees
- 5 fingertip push-ups
- Run 100 meters
- 15 push-ups
- 5 burpees
- 10 clap push-ups
- 5 burpees
- 10 chest slap push-ups
- 5 burpees
- 5 fingertip push-ups
- Run 100 meters
- 10 push-ups
- 5 burpees

- 10 clap push-ups

- 5 burpees

- 10 chest slap push-ups

- 5 burpees

- 5 fingertip push-ups

18. For time

- Run 400 meters

- Burpee broad jump 25 meters

- Walking lunges 25 meters

- Burpee broad jump 25 meters

- Bear crawl 25 meters

- Burpee broad jump 25 meters

- Walking lunges 25 meters

- Burpee broad jump 25 meters

- Bear crawl 25 meters

- Run 400 meters

19. Deck of cards (core variation)

Take a deck of cards; shuffle. Face cards are 10, aces are 11, numbered cards as valued. Flip each card and perform the movement and the number of reps specified. Cycle whole deck.

- Hearts: burpees

- Diamonds: mountain climbers (act)

- Spades: flutter kicks (4 count)

- Clubs: sit-ups

- Jokers: run 400 meters

20. For time

- 50 burpees
- 75 flutter kicks (4 count)
- 100 push-ups
- 150 sit-ups

21. 5 rounds of

- 10 burpees
- 20 box/bench jumps
- 30 push-ups
- 40 squats
- 50 lunges

22. 4 rounds of

- 50 walking lunges
- 50 squats
- Run 400 meters

23. For time

- Run 5 kilometers
- Every 2:00, do 20 push-ups and 20 squats

24. 3 rounds of

- 50 push-ups
- 50 sit-ups
- 50 squats

25. 5 rounds of

- 50 walking lunges
- 15 handstand push-ups

26. For time

- 80 squats
- 10 handstand push-ups
- 60 squats
- 20 handstand push-ups
- 40 squats
- 30 handstand push-ups
- 20 squats

27. 4 rounds of

- 25 lunges
- 50 squats

28. 5 rounds of

- 100 squats
- 20 lunges
- 35 push-ups

29. 5 rounds of

- 50 squats
- 30 handstand push-ups

30. 2 rounds

- Max push-ups 2:00
- Max sit-ups 2:00
- Max flutter kicks 2:00
- Max squats 2:00

31. 3 rounds of

- − 30-yard bear crawl
- − 30-yard inchworm push-up
- − 30-yard burpee jumps

Bonus Chapter 2

How to Automate Shopping for Garage Gym Equipment

What is the best way to shop for home-gym/garage-gym equipment?

A garage sale? The internet? Sporting goods store?

What if I told you that if you implement the super-simple system, laid out in this chapter, you would be able to find great deals on garage gym equipment with no real effort at all?

Seriously, take 10 minutes to try this stuff out, sit back, and let the good deals come to you.

Unless you get lucky at a garage sale (very time consuming), your best bet for finding *great* deals—I mean pennies on the dollar type deals—will be craigslist.

There are just too many people who thought the whole garage gym thing was for them, but then they just didn't like it, probably because they never found a great community of people like here at End of Three Fitness.

But there are two major problems with craigslist: time & timing.

- Time: Because you have to spend a lot of time, day after day checking to see what the latest deals are. Then you may stretch your search to surrounding cities, and cities you have friends in. You could spend hours searching for the right deal.

- Timing: Next, there is the timing issue. Most of us have lives, so we cannot constantly check craigslist for the latest and greatest deal. So, say the perfect deal came along, but you are the sixth person to contact the seller and the item is already gone or the price has gone up. Fail.

Where does that leave us?

Maybe you get fed up and just decide to purchase your garage gym items for quadruple the price, or you could join the twenty-first century.

Let's talk about IFTTT.

IFTTT stands for If This Then That, and helps you automate your e-world. Check out their site if you are unfamiliar at www.ifttt.com.

Well, today IFTTT officially becomes the best way to shop for garage gym equipment!

Step 1: Join IFTTT & use recipe

Sign up for an IFTTT account, if you don't already have one (you should), and search for the recipe: craigslist search. Pretty simple, and it's all free.

Step 2: Search craigslist

Now, go to craigslist and do a search for the item you want. Make sure you are in the right geographical area (duh) and you can even set the price points if you would like.

Once you have done the search, copy the entire URL from craigslist that is in your browser, and proceed to Step 3.

Step 3: Let IFTTT work for YOU

Head back to the recipe at IFTTT and enter the copied URL into the designated space. Rename the e-mail subject line to say, "Garage Gym Deals," and click "use recipe."

BOOM! You're done; IFTTT is now shopping for you.

Yep, you will get an e-mail anytime your search parameters are met—aka, when that perfect deal rolls around that you have been working on, you can get it right away.

Step 4: Repeat

Set up as many alerts for as much gear as you need. Now, you just sit back, relax, and wait for the deals to come to you.

Granted, there is always the chance of the specific deal you want never coming around, but if you live in a big enough area chances are this will work for you.

Give it time—get what you want for the price you want.

Barbell Buyers' Guide

How on earth can you break a barbell?

That was the question I was asking myself while standing in my driveway with, well, a broken barbell.

Years ago, when I purchased my first barbell, I didn't put much thought into type or quality. They are just barbells, right? That thinking (or lack thereof) led to my first barbell breaking within 24 hours of purchase.

Well, with broken barbell in hand I decided it was time to uncover some of the basics as to what makes a good, durable barbell. What I found was that they can range from $200 to $2,000, and they are a little more complicated than your average sporting goods store would have you believe. A barbell serves as the foundation of true strength training. You can get by without a lot of things, but you cannot get by without a barbell.

Buying the right bar will help you to avoid big issues—they can warp, bend, rust, and break. The most common bar mishaps are bending from missed lifts, and sleeves popping off, from more or less, cheap manufacturing. Today, I want to make you an informed consumer of the barbell.

Barbell Basics

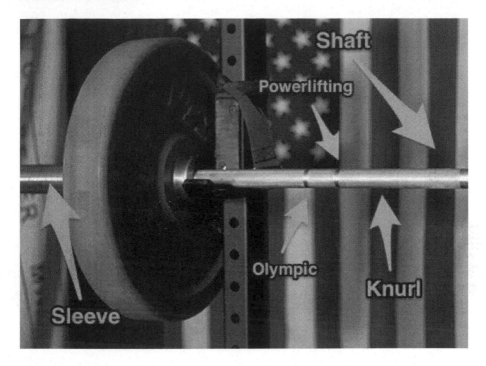

Before you can truly make an informed decision you need to know exactly what a barbell consists of—its "anatomy."

A commonly used barbell has a 28- to 29-mm diameter shaft for men, and 25 mm for women. Barbells come in all shapes and sizes, but the standard length is 7.2 feet for men and about 6.5 feet for women. They weigh about 44 pounds for men (20 kg) and about 33 pounds for women (15 kg).

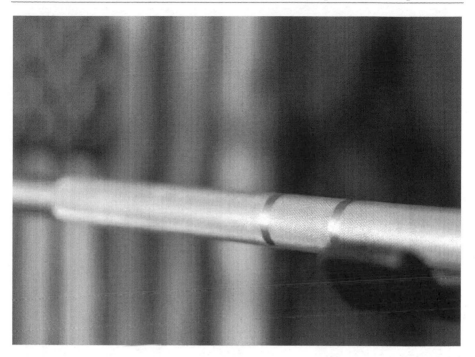

First, you have the bar itself, or shaft. It's put through a machining process to get it to the right length and diameter. On the shaft, you have what is called knurling. Knurling is simply the rough, cross-hatched pattern you see on a barbell. Knurl is very important and is mainly for grip. It is machine pressed and can be extremely rough or smooth, depending on the manufacturer. It is important to feel the bar to get an idea of what you like (unless you buy online—in that case, look at reviews), but most top-end bar manufacturers have a good knurl. Where knurling can differ, even on top-end bars, is where the knurl does and does not exist. Some bars have knurling that extends all the way to the sleeves, and some bars have a gap of no knurling where the bar meets the sleeves. Sometimes bars will have center knurling and sometimes they won't. You have to decide what you want and what you are most comfortable with.

If, say, you like Olympic lifting and you prefer a wide snatch grip, I suggest getting a bar with knurling that extends to the sleeves (if that sentence made no sense, then don't worry about knurling going to the sleeves).

If you are often shirtless or do high-rep front squats and presses (Cross-Fit® anyone?), you may want to go with no center knurling. If you regularly squat heavy weights and need the bar to grip the back, get the center knurling.

Furthermore, the markings on the knurl indicate which type of bar you are using. I recommend a dual-marked bar for general purpose use. However, the outermost marking indicates an Olympic lifting bar and the inner marking indicates a powerlifting bar, and we'll talk more about those in a minute.

It comes down to how it meets your needs and style of fitness.

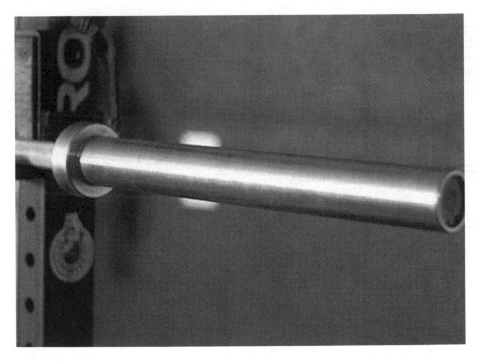

Next, we have the sleeves.

The sleeves are simply where you put the weights. They are created from drawn over mandrel tubing, a machine process that makes the sleeves straight and strong. The biggest thing you are looking for in the sleeves is the rotation, or how the sleeves spin on the shaft. The difference in bearings or bushings isn't that important unless you are extremely picky or a professional lifter. Bushings are a low-friction material placed between the shaft and the sleeve—they are more affordable, and they are what you will find on most bars. Needle bearings spin more smoothly, and are actual bearings between the shaft and the sleeve. Generally, bearings are on the high-end bars. Bushings will save you a lot of money, and work perfectly fine, without having to go high-end. But, if you want the premium, then go bearings. Bearings are better—you aren't paying more without reason—but the difference would only be noticed at the professional and elite levels.

Sleeves are also connected by bolts or snap rings. I will make this one very easy for you. Snap rings only! Stay away from bolts on a bar! Bolts = broken in 24 hours.

Also, know barbells come in many finishes—chrome, zinc, black oxide, unfinished, and even stainless steel—but also know that the finish is primarily an aesthetic preference. Although stainless steel provides an advantage because it is rust and corrosion free, forever.

Barbell Strength

At this point, you already know more than your average gym-goer, but let's make you a true barbell connoisseur.

The strength of a barbell is very important. You need to know the terms I am about to go over, because when you shop for a barbell, this is the information manufacturers will give you. If you have no idea what the numbers are referring to, how do you know what to buy?

Bar strength is reported in three areas: tensile strength, yield strength, and test.

Tensile strength is the maximum load your bar can support without fracturing or breaking. So high tensile strength = good bar. This will be your primary determining factor.

Yield strength is basically how much weight the bar can handle before it will become deformed—that is, it won't return to perfect straightness. Breaking and deformation are very different. Unfortunately, you will be hard-pressed to find a manufacturer that provides yield strength information.

There is also test, meaning the bar has been loaded and tested with weights at which there was no bending or breaking, so the higher, the better. It's best if you can find a manufacturer that will give you a tensile strength rating, which is reported in pounds per square inch (PSI).

Now you know the terminology, but what is a "good" rating? Here is a starting point for the most important factor—tensile strength ratings:

- <150,000 PSI = Eh
- 150,000–175,000 PSI = Good
- 175,000–200,000 PSI = Better
- >200,000 PSI = Best

A bar in the good range is perfectly acceptable and will last a very long time. Considering cost and quality, most people do not need more than the "good" level bar.

If you are getting into sport weightlifting, there are differences in Olympic lifting bars and powerlifting bars:

- Olympic weightlifting bars have more of a whip, or spring, to accommodate the sport.
- Powerlifting bars are very stiff, as powerlifters prefer no surprises or major fluctuations during a big lift.

Barbell Plates

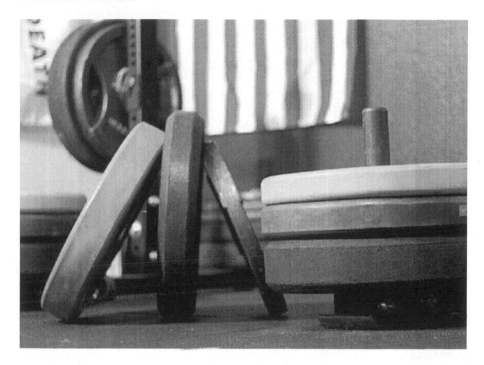

Next, you have to think about plates. Unless you plan on competing at the professional level, plate quality is not as vital as the quality of your barbell.

Price can vary greatly with plates. You can get 300 pounds of iron at a garage sale for $30 or you can spend over $3,000 on a couple hundred pounds of certified competition bumper plates.

The most frequently asked question is whether to purchase bumper plates or iron (metal) plates, and that depends on the type of lifting you plan to do. If you like powerlifting (squat, bench press, and deadlift), then you will be just fine with iron plates. If you are dropping the bar frequently during CrossFit® workouts or practicing the snatch and clean and jerk in Olympic weightlifting, you'll need bumpers.

Personally, I prefer a blend of iron and bumper plates in my arsenal, and I'll explain why and some considerations in just a minute. First, let's talk bumper plates.

When it comes to bumper plates, what you are paying for is the thickness of the plate and how much they bounce when dropped.

Here is a quick breakdown of their categories:

- Black bumpers ($): Thick with a big bounce

- Colored bumpers ($$): Thick with less bounce

- Olympic training bumpers ($$$): Thin and dead bounce

- Competition bumpers ($$$$$$$): Thin and dead bounce + certified weight to the gram

They all should be 450-millimeter disks with a 50-millimeter opening. Economy black bumper plates are going to be good enough for 95 percent of people; 4.9 percent will want/need colored bumpers or Olympic training bumpers, and .1 percent will need certified Olympic competition bumpers. Colored plates generally follow a color coding, and some companies follow the color code of the International Weightlifting Federation, but not all do. The official color coding can be found at the IWF website.

I like to have around 300 pounds of cheap iron plates along with another couple hundred pounds of black bumpers. I use the bumpers for when I am going to be dropping the weight, and I use a combination of iron and bumpers if I am doing a heavy back squat.

You'll be hard-pressed to find bumper plates at a garage sale, so you will need to order them online, but iron plates are a completely different story.

For iron, here's where you use the power of Craigslist to find a lot of weight for pennies on the dollar. People are constantly moving, giving up on at-home fitness, and letting plates sit in their garage and rust. That's a win for us.

Conclusion

Most people are looking for a general, high-quality bar, and there are plenty out there that are suitable for all training and that will last for a long time. So, unless you are planning on becoming an Olympian, I would stay away from the "Cadillac" bars. You can get a good barbell that will meet all of your needs for around $250, and the near-perfect bar for around $500.

That can seem like a lot of money for a barbell, but it is the heart of your training, and you will be using it day in and day out. Don't get a bar that will bend or fail while you are using it.

Get a bar that will last a lifetime. It is an investment in your fitness and your health!

And that, is all you need know about plates, weights, and barbells.

Now, let's start your story differently than mine.

How on earth can this barbell withstand this abuse?

That will be the question you are asking yourself while standing in your driveway with, well, an amazing barbell.

Chapter 27

The Revolution

I couldn't think of a better way to end this book than to show you how crazy I truly am by sharing a poem I wrote in 2011, shortly after I started my own garage gym and End of Three Fitness. The work is based on "The Revolution Will Not Be Televised" poem and song by Gil Scott-Heron.

The Garage Gym Revolution

You will be able to stay home, brother.

You will not be able to plug in, turn on, and cop out.

You will not be able to lose yourself in a sea of fitness machines,

Skip out on real work by talking to your friends,

Because the revolution will not be televised.

The revolution will not be televised.

The revolution will not be brought to you by Nike

In 4 parts without commercial interruptions.

The revolution will not show you pictures of professionals

Drinking a protein shake while wearing "their" shoe.

The revolution will not be televised.

The revolution will not be brought to you by the

Producers of "easy" trying to make fitness what it is not.

There will not be a night and daytime vitamin ad showing

A picture of life that is non-existent.

There will be no television screens attached to robots

Producing an endless cycle of repetitions.

The revolution will not use a cream to get rid of love handles.

The revolution will not be bottled and taken twice daily, because

The revolution will not be televised, Brother.

There will be no secrets and "authority figures" pushing

Jillian Michaels' latest DVD. P90X will fall on deaf ears.

There will be no television network telling us who is the winner

And who is the loser, reported nationally to 50 million viewers.

The revolution will not be televised.

The revolution will not be held on cables and pulleys, yet

Rather by stones and cast iron shapes.

You will not have to worry about who was there before you,

A sweat stain, or a disinfectant wipe.

The revolution will not go better with your favorite TV show.

The revolution will not be programmed into your heart rate monitor.

The revolution will not have a share button.

The revolution will put you in the driver's seat.

The revolution will not be televised, will not be televised,

will not be televised, will not be televised.

The revolution will be no re-run brothers;

The revolution will be live.

Think I'm crazy?

Maybe I am a little crazy.

But maybe you are a little crazy, too.

Welcome to the revolution.

Welcome, Garage Gym Athlete!

Garage Gym Athlete

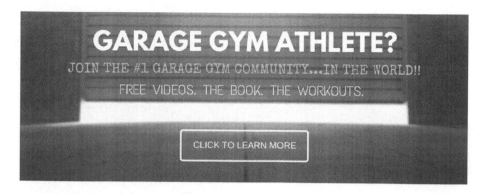

Garage Gym Athlete is made up of three components:

1. Daily Workouts

2. A Thriving Community

3. Training Programs

Garage Gym Athlete provides the highest quality programming at the best price you will find, and it is 100 percent catered to the minimalist garage gym exerciser. Join our community and get stronger, faster and harder to kill!

We have a ton of free resources, projects and workouts you can take advantage of today!

To sign up go to <u>GarageGymAthlete.com</u> and follow the instructions!

Please Review This!

I hope you have enjoyed this *Practical Guide to Training like a Pro, Unleashing Fitness Freedom*, and *Living the Simple Life*.

If this book helped or at least entertained you in any way, all I ask in return is that you take a moment to write an honest, sincere review of this book on Amazon. It will only take a few minutes, and it would help me out more than you can imagine.

About the Author

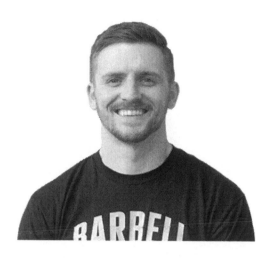

Laying in bed, $100,000 in debt and recovering from an injury stemmed from pulling G's in a high performance aircraft, Jerred Moon realized his dream of becoming a fighter pilot was over – so he returned to his passion for fitness. With no money and still recovering, he started to sketch out how he could build a gym and a business to fully follow his passion of training and coaching. One DIY project at a time, he built a full gym in his garage then started using equations from his aerodynamics and aviation background to develop highly effective strength and conditioning programs. Years passed and his programs gained real traction, his garage gym went from wooden DIY to solid steel, and he built a business which has helped thousands become better versions of themselves—and helped his family crush their debt.

Jerred is a Strength and Conditioning Coach and creator of End of Three Fitness which specializes in simple, effective barbell-centric fitness for the other guy. He's a former Physical Training Leader and Fitness Program Manager within U.S. Air Force Special Operations Command, and he's been featured in WOD Talk Magazine, Sweat RX Magazine, Life Hacker, The Huffington Post, The Art of Manliness, and more. He currently coaches and programs for hundreds of athletes from military operators to stay-at-home mom's. You can connect with Jerred by visiting his website, End of Three Fitness, at <u>EndofThreeFitness.com</u>.

62694546R00120

Made in the USA
Lexington, KY
14 April 2017